C000183901

THE
MADNESS

BY THE SAME AUTHOR

Wounds: A Memoir of War & Love

Road of Bones: The Epic Siege of Kohima 1944

All of These People

Letter to Daniel: Despatches from the Heart

The Bondage of Fear:
A Journey Through the Last White Empire

Season of Blood: A Rwandan Journey

A Stranger's Eye: A Foreign Correspondent's View of Britain

Letters Home

THE MADNESS

A Memoir of War, Fear and PTSD

FERGAL KEANE

WILLIAM
COLLINS

William Collins
An imprint of HarperCollins*Publishers*
1 London Bridge Street
London SE1 9GF

WilliamCollinsBooks.com

HarperCollins*Publishers*
Macken House, 39/40 Mayor Street Upper,
Dublin 1, Ireland D01 C9W8

First published in Great Britain in 2022 by William Collins

1

Copyright © Fergal Keane 2022

Fergal Keane asserts the moral right to be identified
as the author of this work in accordance with the
Copyright, Designs and Patents Act 1988

A catalogue record for this book is
available from the British Library

HB ISBN 978-0-00-842042-0
TPB ISBN 978-0-00-842043-7

All rights reserved. No part of this publication may be
reproduced, stored in a retrieval system, or transmitted,
in any form or by any means, electronic, mechanical,
photocopying, recording or otherwise, without the
prior permission of the publishers.

This book is sold subject to the condition that it shall not, by
way of trade or otherwise, be lent, re-sold, hired out or otherwise
circulated without the publisher's prior consent in any form of
binding or cover other than that in which it is published and
without a similar condition including this condition being
imposed on the subsequent purchaser.

Typeset in Adobe Garamond Pro
Printed and bound in the UK using 100%
renewable electricity at CPI Group (UK) Ltd

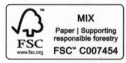

MIX
Paper | Supporting
responsible forestry
FSC™ C007454
www.fsc.org

This book is produced from independently certified FSC™ paper
to ensure responsible forest management.

For more information visit: www.harpercollins.co.uk/green

For Alice

Contents

Prologue: A Trail of Shadows   1

1   The Lying Mirror   13

2   Shapings   26

3   Generations Fighting   45

4   Her Wars   57

5   Hero Child   77

6   Reckonings   90

7   Believing   99

8   Abandoned   113

9   Blackout Boy   122

10   The Fires Are Everywhere   132

11   Terms of Surrender   147

12   Siege   167

13   Old Ground   188

14   Trials   198

15   East   214

16   Trip Wires   234

17   Breakdown   242

18   For Fear of a Dream   256

19   Gathering In   265

     Epilogue: Kinder Voices   275

     A Note on Sources   283
     Acknowledgements   287
     Notes   289

Prologue
A Trail of Shadows

Kyiv, 20 February 2022

I open the curtains and see the light coming up. It will be a beautiful day. There is no cloud. The temperature has risen above zero. Crisp, dry weather with little wind to chill our uncovered faces. A day to walk down Khreshchatyk street and eat in the Turkish restaurant with the view up towards Maidan Square. We sat there last week and saw the demonstrators materialise outside, a long line of them – everyone from far-right nationalists to the local LGBTQ organisations. Only in this part of eastern Europe, this Kyiv, would you see the likes of it. Together, they sang the national anthem – 'Glory to Ukraine' – and then dispersed.

But what is coming? What is coming from across the horizon towards Kyiv, Dnipro, Kramatorsk, Mariupol, Odesa, and all the land that lies in the way of Putin's malign designs?

We have exhausted ourselves with speculation. Every meal is a repeat of the same conversation. The Russia experts among our group think it unlikely that Putin will invade. Or at the worst they think he'll escalate in the east but not try to take Kyiv. There is constant questioning of Allied intelligence which has been warning daily of the invasion threat. How do they really know he is going to attack? My gut says he will not leave this job unfinished and allow a rebellious government to remain in Kyiv. But I waver briefly when the Russians announce they want to de-escalate.

Not for long. Day after day, the armies gather on the border. Pontoon bridges appear. Soon the provocations start in the east. I watch it unfold and think of my friends in the way of the advance. Anatoly and Svetlana, the dear elderly beekeeper and his family who have suffered so much already, live in the path of the Russian army.

Still, see how lovely the light is, the pink glow spreading up the sky from the east. The Russians concealed in the forest see the same dawn. They will be restless. Most soldiers on the eve of battle think of loved ones and home. Or they do their best not to think of what might be lost forever in the days and weeks to come. None know for sure that they won't end up dead or with their guts spilling out, or with some other particularity or combination of anatomical dismemberment, in a muddy field or ruined house.

The Ukrainians facing them see the same light. The people of Bucha and Hostomel and Irpin are heading out to work, or taking their kids to school. I have driven through these places on the way to and from meetings; they are not yet weighted with any significance, just names of places I pass by.

It is five days since I walked in no-man's-land with Major Sergiy Khomenko, who grew up in a border village, whose father was a soldier in Soviet times, and who said he would stand and fight if the Russians came. But nearly every soldier I've ever met said that. Would it be different for him if the columns come rolling down the road, all heavy calibre bullets and rockets, all that insane noise of an army attacking? We were standing near the forest on the border with Belarus, deep snowbound forests that might conceal an army – that probably did: watching us and waiting for its orders to advance. That was a week ago, when I still thought there was a chance, a very small one, that diplomacy might work. But Putin is playing a game and the shrewder of the world leaders know it. His army is coming.

I struggle with myself. To stay or leave? I have made promises: to those I love. To myself. No more front-line war reporting. I also fear my nerves might not be able to take it. Am I asking for another crack-up and hospitalisation? I have said to myself often in the last few years that I cannot endure another breakdown.

But the surge of desire to stay here is so strong. It's in my head, and in the marrow of my bones. The reasons are pouring out. *I'm a reporter, I'm meant for this. History is about to happen, how can I leave this?* I feel the adrenaline pulsing. Going to bed at night part of me wishes to be awoken by explosions so the decision will be taken out of my hands: Kyiv cut off, me unable to leave. Nothing for it but to knuckle down and report the battle for the city. My conscience knows this is an addict's evasion. I watch the sun set on another day without war. I will make my decision soon. Or it will be made for me.

I have been afraid all of my life. Dread still wakes me in the night. It is there to greet me in the morning. It comes at differing velocities. It can be an anxiety that nags all day without a name, or I can be driving down an Irish country road, the sea blue and dreaming on my left, and I have to pull over and sit shaking, hands clasped tight under my armpits, visions of catastrophe swirling in my head, the urge to vomit building, while I struggle to form the words of the Serenity Prayer. A muttering man, dry heaving by the roadside in his late middle age, a sight for no eyes.

God grant me the serenity
To accept the things I cannot change
The courage to change the things I can
And the wisdom to know the difference.

I have been diagnosed with complex post-traumatic stress disorder, a condition arising from exposure to multiple instances of trauma, experienced over a long period. It is regarded as significantly harder to treat than a single traumatic episode. My first PTSD diagnosis was twelve years ago. Since then I have attended numerous sessions of therapy. I have taken courses of anti-depressants, which made me emotionally numb, and physically constipated, but which also prevented me from reaching a stage of desperation where I might harm myself. Despite this, and countless promises to do otherwise, I have gone back to the wars, again and again.

I am also a recovering alcoholic and have been sober for more than twenty years. The bottle was my medication of choice during many of the years I went to the wars. The struggle with alcohol described in this book is an integral part of my attempts, and those of many I know, to escape the pain of PTSD by getting 'out of it', a description of drunkenness that is as accurate a psychological representation of my experience as I've ever read. Out of the pain is where I wanted to be. The consequences of that desire would be unremittingly counterproductive.

Back in January 2019 I declared that I was leaving front-line reporting because of the disorder. The decision was prompted by a nervous collapse the previous summer after a reporting assignment in Sudan. There were expressions of support from the public and other journalists. Under the headline 'We should thank Fergal Keane for bearing witness to unbearable horrors', Suzanne Moore wrote: 'It was tremendously brave, even for a brave man such as the BBC reporter Fergal Keane to talk about Post Traumatic Stress Disorder.'[1]

But I did not feel brave. I especially did not feel I deserved the warm words of the many who sent emails and mentioned me on social media. I was in Rome when the news was made public by the BBC, on a literary pilgrimage, walking the streets in search of the city of Keats and Shelley. I switched my phone off. The welter of comment went away.

The guilt did not.

Why should they praise me, I thought, when I had walked willingly into the darkness for three decades and counting? Numerous therapists over the years had pointed out the dangers to my mental health. Despite the warnings I kept going. Even after experiencing a PTSD breakdown, I found a way to get to Mogadishu, at that point the most dangerous city on earth.

After that my therapist Cristina seemed to lose patience with me: 'What the hell were you doing in Somalia?' she asked. 'I mean honestly! What about your promise?' I had never heard her so animated before. 'You know where this leads! You will go down again.'[2]

'I should have stopped after Belfast,' I said to her. But we both knew I could not have stopped back then, not being who I was.

I wrote about some of the events in this book nearly twenty years ago in a memoir. At that point I did not yet have a diagnosis for what felt like a kind of madness. I sense, in the prose of my younger years, if not evasions, then certainly an inability to go to the heart of my matter: the paradox of a man who suffered from acute trauma but who repeatedly placed himself in traumatic situations. Much has happened to me since in my experience of

PTSD, and in treatment of the condition more generally. Here I hope is a narrative informed by experience and some painful lessons.

My subjects are motive, consequence, and recovery. I am afraid of the self-exposure involved here, yet I know that such fear is my enemy. It is what keeps me trapped in pain and seeking to escape it by going back to the war, the ultimate land of forgetting.

I will try to explain why I went back again and again, long after the damage was apparent. There are caveats. I was not somebody simply addicted to war. Since childhood I had a consuming curiosity about the world. My favourite subject at school was history. That passion has remained undimmed. I also had an instinctive loathing of bullies and wanted to challenge them and to record the voices of those who suffered because of the decisions of powerful men. I felt privileged to be able to be able to work as a journalist, especially in those parts of the world where prison and murder were used to silence locals who spoke out.

Such high-minded imperatives are easy to offer and to have accepted as expiation for a life lived on the edge. They were a staple of war reporters' memoirs – along with the thrilling tales of derring-do and poignant depictions of the suffering of strangers, reported back by the wounded soul who goes to hell so that the viewers, listeners and readers don't have to. All that is fine, if that is as far as you want to go in the question of motivation.

But in my case, there was also something much harder to accept and to explain to others: an irresistible compulsion to be where the night was darkest. In the words of Sheridan Le Fanu, the path I chose in life was 'drawing me interiorly into hell'.[3] I worked in places where death and serious injury were not abstractions. For all my experience and training, tragic consequences were often just a moment's bad luck away.

In my BBC office I look across the desk at Frank Gardner, paralysed from the waist down by a gunman in Saudi Arabia in the same attack in 2004 that killed our cameraman colleague Simon Cumbers. Near Frank is Stuart Hughes who lost his lower leg after stepping on a landmine in Iraq in 2003. The same blast killed Iranian photojournalist Kaveh Golestan. On the wall behind me is a photo of my friend Kate Peyton, murdered in Somalia in a drive-by shooting in 2005, and whose body I was called to identify. Kate was a gentle person, a beautiful singer. She had recently found love and adopted her partner's daughter. Neither Simon nor Kaveh nor Kate were compulsively driven to seek the dangers of the battlefield. But war took them anyway.

There are numerous others I knew who died on assignment or came home with wounds of the body and mind. Very few, save friends, families, lovers, remember the dead war journalists. The world moves on. In my sad and anxious times I think of them and berate myself: *You have nothing to complain about. You have your legs and arms. You are alive ...* I remember them when anniversaries roll around or old friends gather and we talk about the past, or when I wake at night and pace the flat.

To speak of symptoms: I get angry too easily. I overreact to any situation or statement that threatens my security. I am constantly on my guard. I wear myself out with my murmuring, ever-present anger, the struggle to keep it from rising and making a misery of the lives of others. The struggle is not only with fear, nightmares, flashbacks, intrusive images and memories – the panoply of post-traumatic stress – but with recurring periods of deep depression. My psychological maladies do not sit neatly in one box. There is for me, as well, a reckoning with the erosion of belief in myself as a moral person that deepened every time I walked away from those who were suffering and whom I felt powerless to help. The battle between who I was, and who I wished to be, was endless. The adversary, as Carl Jung put it, was 'none other than "the other in me"',[4] or if I can put it in less elegant terms: if there is a darkness in you, an obsessive, a compulsive, fucked up part of you, war will find it and carry you to places most people would never dream of going. And it will keep you going.

Most war in my lifetime has mutated into some new misery. Can anybody calculate what it does to the human spirit to witness the savagery and cynicism of humankind over more than thirty years, and to keep going back for more? The phrase they use for it nowadays is *moral injury*, and it is a recurring theme of this book. There is no unseeing.

The sitting room of the home of John O'Neill senior, Ligoniel, north Belfast in the weeks after the murder of his son, John junior, who was lured into a loyalist drinking club in March 1986 and then taken outside, dragged to a lonely spot near a stream, and beaten and stabbed to death. His body was identified by his red hair, the same hair as his father and mother. John senior tells me how he went to the scene a few days after the killing and called out to his child. The place was in loyalist territory but the father felt no fear. He was beyond that. There was rain falling. All he could think of was the loneliness of his son's end …

… The mother washing the blood of her murdered husband from a doorstep in Tokoza, the pink of the soapy water and the stillness of her children looking at me through the window of their little house. Witness, stranger, curator of intimate agonies.

... The village in Sri Lanka where the guerrillas beheaded
several children, leaving the bodies lying in a row. When we
found the survivors they could barely speak but they held up
to us a photograph of the dead. My mind cannot find now
the picture of the mutilated children, but I do see – as clear as
if it were yesterday – the fingers of a boy playing with water as
it flowed from a tap in the makeshift refugee camp.

I was not conscious then of how these scenes might replay again
and again in my mind in the years to come. I knew nothing about
post-traumatic stress disorder as a specific medical condition. I
was aware of shellshock in the Great War and had seen the
Vietnam films with their clichés of thousand-yard stare veterans.
The idea that the mental disturbances of war might extend to
journalists seems obvious now, but study of the subject is comparatively recent.

In the first major study of war reporters and PTSD, published
in the *American Journal of Psychiatry* in 2002, the researchers
found that 25 per cent of the sample group experienced PTSD.
The authors noted that 'war journalists have significantly more
psychiatric difficulties than journalists who do not report on war.
In particular, the lifetime prevalence of PTSD is similar to rates
reported for combat veterans, while the rate of major depression
exceeds that of the general population.'[5]

I have some colleagues who have witnessed as much horror as I
have, and not been immobilised, or even obviously affected, as I
was by trauma. Why me and not them? A question that has gone
around and around in my head and leads me back always to the
conclusion that I am flawed, weak, not the person they are. There
is a more compassionate, and accurate, explanation: the individual mind is magnificent in its complexity and people can vary

enormously in their responses to events. What I write here is the story of my own experiences. The statistical evidence, however, supports a picture of wider traumatic impact among those who are journalist witnesses.

I also know, through my friendships, through conversations late at night on the front lines, that many who specialise in reporting conflict zones are survivors of childhood trauma, having grown up in environments shaped by addiction, abuse, neglect. It is no coincidence, I believe, that we find ourselves drawn to the world's disintegrating places. The tension and the sorrow represent something familiar, challenges that we were prepared for by our experiences as children, the hook that pulled me back endlessly.

The journey I describe here goes far back, beyond my years as a reporter in zones of conflict. Childhood in a home made fearful by alcoholism was the foundation of my trauma. I remember a counsellor asking me once: 'What would you say to the young Fergal?' And I replied, with barely a pause, 'I'd tell him to fuck off out of it while he still had the chance.' Escape was in my head from way back.

I believe that PTSD existed in me long before I ever set foot on a battlefield. The specialists call it 'amygdala hijacking', where 'the psychic imprinting of PTSD results in changed brain chemistry; the amygdala triggers the nervous system and panic, and prolonged panic may result in permanent panic'.[6]

This book is a story of living in fear – from the wars of the late twentieth and early twenty-first centuries, back all the way to eruptions at home, the violence that pervaded our schoolrooms, the bullies in the playground who laughed at my facial twitches and how I jumped at the slightest noise or disturbance. A recurring private terror was that my family would fall apart, and I would be taken and placed in one of the country's notorious industrial schools. The names Letterfrack, Daingean, Artane – the industrial schools where boys were brutalised – were whispered in dread in the Ireland of those days. Looking back, I realise that this was not a remotely realistic prospect; I had a wide circle of loving relatives who would have cared for me without a moment's hesitation. But what does the small child know when his entire being has become hyper-sensitised to threat? In my child's mind, I believed that neither home nor state was a safe place to be.

Some emerge from dysfunctional homes with an overwhelming desire for routine. They avoid conflict. I came out of childhood with a determination to prove that I could be brave. I was also determined to be seen and heard. My validation came through the praise and recognition of others.

But beyond the impact of my lived experience, there is another important question that forms part of the story of PTSD that I describe here: is it possible that some of the trauma experienced by previous generations of my family might have affected me? The study of intergenerational trauma – where genetics, social science and history intersect – looks to the potential influence of past events on current generations.

History is my constant preoccupation. In every conflict I have covered I have taken care to try to know the longer story. History shapes the individual mind as much as it does the borders of nations. Famine, Revolution, Civil War – all influenced how my forebears saw the world. This is why the story of my people in Ireland is described in this story of PTSD. I grew up in an era where the mentally ill were stigmatised, an environment that made me determined to avoid psychiatrists and hospitals. I didn't manage that, and this book is the story of why.

This book is written in memory of those who died in the wars, and for those broken in body and mind. I have taken care here to write what I remember of my experiences and of what it felt like to be in the places I have been, from my childhood to the front lines. It is not within my rights to describe how others who were close to me experienced those times, or how they were affected by the consequences of my choices. This is not to shy away from responsibility but to respect privacy. Their experiences belong to them.

There is no tidy tale of redemption here. The long struggle with myself does not serve up a reassuring narrative of suffering, self-discovery, and *closure*. The word is absurd. We do not open a door into the past, sweep the room clean and then lock it forever. The dead stay dead. The mind is not a hard drive to be wiped clean.

I write to make sense of things for myself, but in the reaction to my stepping down from my job as Africa Editor, and to the film I made about PTSD, I was struck by how my experience resonated with others. I had numerous emails and messages asking me to keep talking and writing on the subject. This book then is also for others struggling with post-traumatic stress, and for those of you who are children of the numberless small wars fought out in dysfunctional homes, whose suffering is so often silent, and for whom there will never be any medals or awards to recognise the heroism your survival has demanded. You are not alone.

1

The Lying Mirror

...
Shaken out long and clear upon the hill,
No merry note, nor cause of merriment,
But one telling me plain what I escaped
And others could not ...

...
Speaking for all who lay under the stars,
Soldiers and poor, unable to rejoice.

'The Owl', Edward Thomas (1917)[1]

An owl is calling from the trees at the bottom of the drive. It must be nesting between the hospital and the tennis club. So close, so clear the music, that it passes through the open window and fills my room every night. There are foxes too, though the call of the vixen disturbs me. It is too close to the shrieking of a tormented body.

The hunting is good in this westerly suburb. There is woodland and tall meadow grass, a brook that fills with frogs and small fish in the summer and an abundance of well-stocked rubbish bins.

13

For a few minutes the owl's sharp call lifts me from my despair. The emotional mess that has brought me here is pushed to the margin. The window will not open fully – this to keep the patients from bounding free in the dead of night – but if I go down on my knees I can smell river and grass nearby and, carried on the breeze, the city smells of cars and buses and restaurants. Every fifteen minutes or so a train rattles across Barnes Common, going to Waterloo or taking the last travellers to the outer reaches of Surrey and Hounslow. I imagine the normal lives beyond the walls. The children safely asleep in their beds. Couples making love with the window open against the heat.

I hear Robert Lowell's words about the 'sick spirit' on a summer night. To paraphrase that great laureate of the misbegotten: my head is unwell.

This is not my first stay in a psychiatric hospital. I had my first breakdown at the age of twenty-nine. It began at Heathrow Airport, as I waited to board a flight to South Africa in 1990, where I was taking up the position of Southern Africa correspondent for the BBC – a job I had long dreamed of, yet for months before I had been consumed by a sense of impending doom.

Waiting for the South African Airways flight to Johannesburg I went to make a phone call home. I felt disoriented. After years of such attacks, I can see now that the onset of a bout of mental illness is always signalled by forgetfulness, a sense that the world is speeding up and I am unable to keep pace, or I am outside the world trying to get back in. I began to cry on the call and was eventually unable to speak. I said goodbye and went to the check-in. I felt ice-cold waves washing down me. These were the triggering of my body's fight-or-flight response – the release of adrenaline into the bloodstream to meet a threat.

Then panic. I discovered I'd left my money belt and tickets at the phone kiosk. I raced back to find them already gone.

The waves of anxiety increased. The airline found my booking on the computer and allowed me to board. The BBC said not to worry. Just get on the flight. They would report the money stolen. I boarded and sat in the middle of a row of four seats. For eleven hours, south towards Africa, I fought the panic. I wept and shook. My fellow passengers were perplexed. The air crew were sympathetic but concerned. Was I going to erupt in a mad fury and alarm everybody else? I reassured them that my troubles were my own. I would not bother anybody else. I moved between my seat and the toilet. I wept, vomited, wrapped my arms under my armpits to try and limit the shaking. But every time it seemed as if I might fall asleep, the panic returned.

Then the plane developed an engine fault. It shook and groaned. I did not have the mental energy to worry about the possibility of crashing. So deep was my own panic that I could not grasp the possibility of a genuine existential threat. We were diverted to Namibia and landed safely. There was a wait in the desert heat at Windhoek, then on to Johannesburg and the hotel. The terror was getting worse.

I had never experienced mental anguish with a such a powerful physical force. The panic created a distorted world in which I was alone, bereft of love and family and friends; a man for whom there was no future, falling down a tunnel, nothing to grab hold of as I flew, and knowing there was no bottom to it, just endless fear. The hotel room began to spin. My heart raced. I threw up again. I phoned loved ones. I try to imagine now how much it must have worried them.

I went outside and roamed the streets. The terror drove me on, through a shopping arcade where I stalked through the crowds. It occurred to me to try and find a doctor's surgery. I knew I was in trouble. Nothing on this scale had happened before. I asked some people for directions or advice, but I remember very little of that part of the afternoon. I went outside again. This was October and the thunderstorms of the southern summer were starting. The rain came down and I was soaked. At one point I weaved precariously through traffic. An elderly woman saw my distress and guided me back to the hotel where I asked the hotel receptionist to call a doctor. The half hour or so that it took him to reach me was terrifying. I was convinced that at any moment I would cease to exist: my heart would stop, or I would choke. The doctor arrived – good-humoured, kind-hearted, a man in his sixties – and spoke words of reassurance. He gave me an injection of sedative and urged me to sleep.

I lay down but the room kept spinning. The injection did not work. Several hours later I called him to come back. An hour or more passed while he dealt with some other patients at his clinic. Second time around he decided I should be admitted to hospital. Before that he gave me another, stronger injection. Gradually the panic sank beneath the sedative fog. I recall a journey by car, through another thunderstorm, to the hospital. Everything was happening outside of me. Forms were filled in. Calls made to my doctor and therapist in Ireland. I woke up the following day in a hospital bed and learned that I was going home. The BBC had been informed and decided I should take sick leave. They would hold my job for me until I was well enough to go back to South Africa. I was too terrified and exhausted to feel a sense of failure. That would come later.

It took weeks for the panic to abate. I depended on tranquillisers to get through the day until sleeping tablets took over at night. I chain-smoked.

Gradually I weaned myself off medication. I went to therapy. I was told I had 'a serious abandonment issue related to childhood', and that at moments of great personal stress this would rise up and overwhelm me in the form of panic attacks. I was told to connect with my 'inner child'. This was all true, but there was much more happening in my head.

In those days nobody in Ireland was talking about post-traumatic stress disorder, much less the possibility that it was something that could develop in childhood. My focus was on getting well enough to get back to South Africa. No therapist could have convinced me that heading to places where people might be killed in front of me was a bad idea.

My ambition returned. The breakdown in the winter of 1990/91 was ascribed to depression. Not likely to recur, I assured my editors. In any event, the news business forgets quickly. Over the years I would learn that as managers moved on, so too did any institutional memory of the detail of my psychological troubles. This has changed, as more and more journalists present with psychological problems. I was soon in the thick of the biggest international news story of the period, watching a recently released Nelson Mandela lead Black South Africans towards free elections. Professionally I became successful. South Africa launched me into the consciousness of the radio-listening public. The breakdowns would recur for the next twenty-five years.

But there is something definitive about the collapse I experience in the summer of 2018 – a conviction that I cannot ever again endure the pain which has brought me to hospital in west London on this night of calling owls and stifling heat. I am too tired, too old to go on living with the self I have embodied until now. I am morbidly fearful. Like Chekhov's doctor hurrying through the rain to conduct an autopsy, I feel 'a strange oppressive dread … as if some misfortune were about to overwhelm me'.[2]

My children are asleep in another part of the city. My arms ache to hold them. My stomach churns in shame. *You have brought this on yourself. All your wars have led to this.* I know that this is not how they see me. I know logically that their love is generous and boundless. But my mind is not operating logically.

A memory.

It is sometime in the middle of March 2003, the night before I depart for the Iraq War. I have pushed hard to go to the front. I will be a 'unilateral', trying to report the fighting with a small team, away from the 'embedded' reporters already waiting in the desert with the armies of the West.

My head is far away already. The party scenes are happening to other people in another world. I need to be gone from here before I weaken and decide I won't go at all. I find my brother-in-law and ask if he will come and walk with me. We have only walked a few yards when I break down and tell him I am afraid I will not come back. This fear has been on my back all day. He embraces me and I lean in to the comfort of his words: 'You always come back. You have a lucky star over you.'

I leave before the house is awake.

I went to the war. I came back. I went away again. I kept going to the wars.

The night nurse puts her head around the door. 'It's hot tonight,' she says. She waits for me to speak. I nod and she retreats. She is from Zimbabwe and, a few days previously, when I had begun to emerge from the dead weight of temazepam, we spoke of places we knew in common: Marondera, Chinhoyi, Rusape. They were some of my roads. I am eager that she likes me. That anybody would like me. But I have no wish to speak tonight.

The nurses are discreet here. After the first few days of being watched I am left to my own devices. The checks slip away, from every hour to every few hours. Once or twice in the deep night my door will open, and a nurse's head will peep inside. A moment, and then gone. I sleep lightly, but I don't resent the interruptions. There is a profound comfort to this sense of being watched over.

The other patients are asleep, or they lie awake in their own anguish. Occasionally somebody gets up. A room door will open, followed by footsteps in the corridor, a heavy shuffle to the nurses' station and then back and the door closes again. Our little wing is a lost colony.

It is a quiet period. There are only a few patients on the men's ward. We meet in the communal kitchen for meals. Occasionally we smoke a cigarette on the lawn outside. The days are filled with long silences.

I do not make friends. That's the thing about repeat visits to hospitals of the mind. You become, as it were, a bit of a 'professional headcase'. Do what is needed to get through and get out. I do not seek companionship or friendships. They involve too many questions.

What could I say to give comfort to those on their first stay? *Don't worry, you'll be as good as new in no time?* Maybe they will, maybe they won't. I cannot offer comfort where at this moment I can find none myself.

I need to sleep, to let my beaten brain rest. I am marking time. I accept there is no cure that will send me bouncing back into the world. *Learn to live with it or die from it. Do not expect a 'Hallelujah Chorus' of redemption.*

It is still deep night. I look at my phone. It's just after two. I go to ask the nurse for more medication. She says that I've already had my prescription for the night. I tell her that I am afraid to sleep because of my nightmares and if I do not sleep, I will become desperate. This is emotional blackmail. It is also the truth. I do not want to suffer. She relents and gives me a second small dose of zolpidem. It takes half an hour for the drug to work and then I am gone.

Sleep is a fever. I wake sodden after two hours. My mouth tastes of rust. A breeze has come, it blows through the half-open window and plays across my body. My T-shirt clings cold to my skin. The questions multiply. *How will this affect my children? What will happen to my job? … What if I can no longer provide? If this keeps happening, then what?*

I remember that there is some Xanax in my bag. I should have handed them over on arrival but was too afraid of being over-whelmed by my anxiety. Call them insurance. A swig from my water bottle and down go the two tablets. I wait for the numb-ness, the delicious recumbence, and I am afraid no more. I am passing 'like night, from land to land …'[3]

When I wake in the early morning there is a lightening in the sky beyond the trees. I know that if I lie here the rumination will begin again.

The night staff have finished their shift. I brace myself for the cheery good mornings of the day team. 'I'd like to go out and smoke,' I say.

I sign out and they buzz the door open. I am free to go into the garden and light a cigarette and stand among the trees. The glow of dawn, of what will become a hot summer day, is visible through the branches. There is a crow shadowing a squirrel. It was Fred Scott who pointed the pair out to me when he came to visit the other day.*

Fred is my brother from the wars. He's been bombed and wounded, kidnapped in Syria, and a lot more. I remember when he was taken in Syria in the days when ISIS was beginning its rise, and where soon the extremists would be parading their victims in orange jumpsuits and then slitting their throats for the cameras. I dreaded that my friend would one day appear on the internet, forced into a denunciation of his country before being murdered. Then came the phone call telling me he was free and on his way to Beirut. That night he called and told me the story of what had happened.

A guide had sold out the team to criminals just after they crossed the border from Lebanon into Syria. Instead of going to a zone controlled by more moderate rebels, they were taken to a village and locked in a basement, awaiting onward sale to ISIS or Al-Qaeda. The four men in the BBC team figured there were two choices: die gruesomely at the hands of the extremists or try to escape. Among the team was a mutual friend of Fred and mine, a former SAS trooper who now acted as a security advisor in war zones. With his guidance, a plan was hatched. The four overpowered the man guarding them and raced out into the streets of the village. By extraordinary good fortune they ran into a patrol of the Free Syrian Army and were rescued.

* Frederick Bradshaw Scott, native of San Diego, war cameraman and comrade of more than twenty-five years, veteran of almost every war there has been since 1989 when he started to work for the BBC.

I clash with Fred sometimes, a collision of 'strong' personalities. We are neither of us the type to take a step backward under pressure. Our first scrap was back in 1995 when we were filming on a roadside in Afghanistan and a Taliban jet – 'Mullahs in Migs' Fred called them – came swooping out of a clear sky. I ran for the nearest ditch, followed by Fred.

'Where's my fucking tripod?' he screamed at me.

The tripod was still standing in the middle of the road, abandoned in terror by me.

'Fuck your tripod, it will survive,' I shouted back.

An image from the following day:

We are hiding in an orchard outside Kabul. The Mujahedin of Ahmed Shah Masoud are laying siege to the city. Mortar fire goes back and forth. A one-legged commander boasts of his contempt for the fundamentalist warriors on the other side of the line. (He lost his leg to the Soviets in the 1980s.) A pickup comes racing along the road from the direction of Kabul: gunmen sit along its edges, and on its bed is the body of a young fighter. A sheet has been drawn over him, but I can still see bare feet – so pale, almost translucent, an unearthly colour, flesh drained entirely of life. When Fred approaches with his camera, the Mujahedin get angry. Rifles are pointed. We mumble words of contrition and back away.

Fred is the comrade I trust most when it comes to hospital. I know he will never repeat a word of what he sees or what I tell him. War breeds madness but also bonds of loyalty. Like so many of us, he is the child of a 'broken' family. He grew up in San Diego among the surfers and the skateboarders but was always too eager for experience and knowledge to settle for the life of a Californian beach boy, or to grind his days out in an office.

Fred has one of the most agile minds I know, filled with knowledge about any amount of unusual things – like the iron content of certain mountains in central Africa; the Spanish conquest of what is now Texas; great recipes for guacamole and stuffed peppers; and the relationship between squirrels and crows. Fred has his own wounds of war. But his stories take me out of myself.

'Watch now,' he says, 'how the crow shadows the squirrel because he's waiting to see where the stash of nuts and stuff is hidden. The minute the squirrel vanishes the crow will steal it. No matter how many times this happens the squirrel doesn't get what's happening. The poor, dumb fucker goes on doing the same thing.' At this we each pause a beat and laugh together.

I will be here for another three weeks according to my consultant. I have known Dr Niall Campbell for around fifteen years.* He was here when I first came in to get sober. Dr C, as he is known, is an Irishman, a Ballymena Protestant, who has done me the great favour of treating me like an adult while recognising the wounded boy within. He understands war and trauma and the history from which I emerge: as a young doctor during the Troubles, he was caught up in an IRA bomb attack in London.

'Will it ever get better?' I ask him.

'It has before,' he replies, 'it will again.'

This afternoon, after a session of group therapy – there was only myself, a mother in the depths of post-natal depression, and

---

* Dr Niall Campbell, consultant psychiatrist, Priory Hospitals. A native of County Antrim, and specialist in the treatment of addiction and trauma.

a somnambulant young man from my ward – I go into the garden to lie in the sun. A few alcoholics from the rehabilitation unit are kicking a ball around. They keep to themselves. The camaraderie of the addicts must not be risked by mingling with the traumatised, depressed and otherwise tormented. They need large doses of hope and none of my bunch are brimming with that substance: we are the Glums; they are the Wine Glums. This is the terminology I remember from my own stint in rehab twenty years ago. Then I was in *their* place, crawling to hotel minibars in the middle of the night to stop myself shaking and dry heaving. I got sober here and I have stayed sober all these years despite all that's come at me, that I've put myself through. In the bleak early hours, I repeat to myself: *That must count for something. Mustn't it?*

Planes pass overhead on their way to and from Heathrow. I light cigarette after cigarette. The alcoholics go to their therapy. The teenage children from the eating disorder unit appear, chaperoned by a nurse and a therapist, and undertake their afternoon walk around the boundary of the hospital. One girl is pushed in a wheelchair. They seem to me, children of a lying mirror: it reflects what must still be starved away. Such brave journeys, I think. Each one of them.

I am waiting for Cristina to return from holidays.* For me she is the best trauma therapist in this place and knows all of my truths. Years ago, she warned me to come away from the wars. Once again, I will ask her to help me untangle the mess into which I have driven myself.

The BBC are supportive. There is no rush back to work. I read into that an imprecation: *Please, really, really take the time it will*

---

* Cristina Garcia-Llavona, psychotherapist specialising in the field of PTSD for over twenty-five years.

take to get better. I have been given a peaceful space in which to go back, far, to the beginning and the battering of a mind that began when I could first hear, then see, and be afraid.

2

Shapings

As long ago when they would take the light
And leave the little child who would have prayed,
Frozen and sleepless at the thought of death.

Sara Teasdale[1]

It hurts to look back with clear eyes to the boy I was. I see him scared. Twisting in bed. Watching the beams from the lights of cars on Ashdale Road, counting out the time between them, until the night falls away and it is light, and safe to sleep.

That boy, who is a boy and not a boy. He is a grown man too, a hunter in a dark forest, armed against all threats, always one step ahead of whatever might be coming. He can turn on a pin; nobody on this street thinks faster on his feet. An expert seducer too – manipulating and scheming to win affection. But under this always the churning fear. The moments of peace are getting fewer. Soon the ceasefire will break, things will be broken, voices raised, doors slammed. Somewhere someone will be weeping. He knows who he really is, the little shitbag. This deserver of all the ruin that he sees. Shame sweats out of his pores. That is only right, he deserves nothing less. Who could love such a creature, who allows his family to fall apart?

Why can I not hold this boy and be kind? Why do I judge him, and who he is becoming?

The baby can see, hear, touch, smell her. She sings old songs, some that her father once sang: 'O Mary this London's a wonderful place, with people here working by day and by night.'[2] They are home all day together. He catches the sound of her words as they sail through the air. He falls asleep to her voice. Hers is the heart that beats against the ear of her first-born, the echo of generations.

And then there are other sounds: chairs, windows, dishes, breaking. A man's voice – loud. The heart pumps fast as cortisol crashes through my tiny body. I see things: sudden movements I cannot understand.

I believe that my post-traumatic stress disorder started in my mother's womb. This is by no means a speculative conclusion: science tells us that from eighteen weeks the baby starts to hear and becomes increasingly sensitive to sound. Nearly sixty years later I still startle and flinch at sudden noises.

My baby's brain is an intricate, malleable thing, bristling with a hundred trillion neural connections. By six months of age my amygdala recognises specific threats. This almond-shaped section of brain, measuring two and a half centimetres across, evolved to prepare humans for fight or flight, to keep our distant forebears alive.

I learn early the registers of my parents' emotions, the difference between love and anger. By the time of my first birthday, I know instinctively that the world, my world, the only world the baby knows, can be a dangerous place. Things happen in my infant brain that shape me forever. As one scholar puts it: 'Through the decades, almost every neurotransmitter system and a multitude of brain regions have been implicated as mediating or impacted by early life experiences.'[3]

So what if, contrary to what I grew up believing, the unhappiness and dysfunctional behaviours that beset me were not caused by mental or 'moral weakness' but are rooted in the science of my brain? This isn't an alibi for who I became, the screw-ups and the addictions, or the choices I made. It is context.

Scientists at Harvard University have concluded that trauma experienced early in childhood can create a vulnerability to depression, alcoholism, drug addiction, and also heart attacks and strokes: 'Extreme exposure to toxic stress can change the stress system so that it responds at lower thresholds to events that might not be stressful to others, and, therefore, the stress response system activates more frequently and for longer periods than is necessary, like revving a car engine for hours every day. This wear and tear increases the risk of stress-related physical and mental illness later in life.'[4] I have already experienced alcoholism and depression. Now that I am in my sixties, I fear the possibility of the physical consequences of that childhood stress, compounded by the demands on my body of decades roving the world's front lines.

I was born on 6 January 1961, while my parents were temporarily sojourning in London. They had arrived from Ireland the previous October so my father, Eamonn, could take up the role of understudy in a major West End production of J. M. Synge's *The Playboy of the Western World*. The Playboy is a rural labourer who arrives in a remote village in County Galway bragging that he has killed his abusive father. His masculine bravado wins the love of a local beauty who showers him with praise: 'You should have had great people in your family … and you a fine, handsome young fellow with a noble brow … it's the poets you are like – fine, fiery fellows with great rages when their temper's aroused.'[5]

A week later, after the play's run had finished, the young couple and their infant son took the boat from Holyhead to Dublin. Ireland was where my father was more likely to find work on stage, TV and radio; there would be plenty of offers for a man with his talent. My mother set her face against failure. She was twenty-six years old, a decade younger than her husband, and still believed that she might heal him of his alcohol addiction. The illusions forged in love, and later in desperation, are strong. 'How young we were, how ignorant,' the poet Evan Boland wrote, 'how ready to think the only history was our own.'[6]

Alcohol and its dysfunctions permeated the world of my father's childhood. His father, Bill, had a weakness for the bottle, but he was not overthrown by it in the same manner as my father. Drink ran through Keane veins as far back as we could trace. My father once told me that a long ago relative had died after falling from a bridge drunk, believing he was riding a horse. That might have been true, or not. My father was a teller of stories big and small. They were his way of taking painful realities and distilling them into material to raise a laugh, a crutch to move from scene to scene. There were stories too of relatives who had squandered hopes of acquiring land, or of job promotion through their fondness for whiskey and porter. In those days they might say of an alcoholic: *He is a martyr to the drink … He drank the farm. He drank the business. Or, he is a lighting demon with drink in him. He's a Holy Terror …*

In Listowel, the town in north Kerry where my father grew up, it was said the town had a licensed premises for every week of the year, each with its own regular clientele. My memory of those places is of a secretive world of male forgetting. The doors were closed, and the world of women, children, unemployment, dead-end jobs, grocery bills and responsibilities shut out.

There had been public houses in Listowel for over four centuries, through rebellions, the Great Famine, the Irish Revolution and Civil War, thriving despite the determined attempts of the priesthood to preach temperance. In the words of a clerical chronicler: 'Irishmen, panting for enjoyment, which was denied them in its legitimate form – the enjoyment of education – turned in their ignorance to drink, and drink brought its concomitants: ruin, misery, and degradation.'[7] The famed Father Theobald Matthew, 'Apostle of Temperance', passed through Listowel on his way to Tralee. A newspaper reported that 'on St. Stephens day a procession of two hundred reclaimed or restrained drunkards marched in procession through Tralee, and made a very orderly and creditable appearance'.*

I would sometimes go and find my father in the pub and sit with him, the self-nominated child hostage against the long bender. In this way, anxiety and vigilance became engrained in me. I was becoming a 'rescuer' who believed it was not only his responsibility but within his power to save someone from destruction. 'The days of our childhood together were steep steps into a collapsing mind,' wrote the American poet Claudia Rankine. 'It looked like we rescued ourselves, were rescued. Then there are these days, each day of our adult lives.'[8]

I drank my lemonade while the men spoke of politics, football, horses, the air thick with the fug of cigarette smoke and

---

* Father Theobald Matthew was a Catholic priest from a landowning family who launched a movement for total abstinence from alcohol, which at its height in the mid-eighteenth century claimed up to 3 million adherents, roughly half the adult population of Ireland.

porter. In this society the man who didn't drink was an oddity. I was conscious of the change that came over my father with each passing drink. He would be irritated and nervous before the first. Then charming, reciting poems and holding the circle of drinkers in the palm of his hand. But somewhere around the fourth or fifth pint he would be enveloped by melancholy. I would sit worrying that he'd embarrass us both by telling the stories of the wrongs done to him, or that he would fall asleep, and I would not be able to get him home. Other men would make their excuses and leave to go home for their tea. These people cared for my father as one of their own. This was his town, and nobody wanted to see him make a 'show' of himself. Most men had a stop button when it came to drink. I gradually understood that my father did not. Sometimes he'd manage to last a week or even a whole fortnight, once or twice when I was a child he went several months without it. But when he did drink, he could not stop.

As a child, my aunts and uncles told me, Eamonn Keane was handsome, clever, charismatic, troubled, and angry – his childhood furies were legendary. He craved the love and attention of his mother, who was beset by the challenge of running a house with seven children, several in-laws who lived with the family, and the struggle with her husband's drinking. My father absorbed the tensions of his home. He was also traumatised at school by a notorious priest who mercilessly thrashed the boys in his care for infractions, real or imagined.

Decades after he had left St Michael's College in Listowel, Eamonn would share with me his memories of being beaten by Father David O'Connor. The school's official website, no less, describes St Michael's as a place where – in my father's time – the teachers were known 'as much for their strict discipline as for their love of learning'.[9] My father's brother, John B., could never forget the abuse he endured at Fr O'Connor's hands: 'The brutality of one particular teacher is something I will never quite forget. I still have the marks from beatings I received on countless occasions, but others suffered as much as I.'[10]

There was a prevailing mentality in Ireland then that a good beating never harmed anyone. Frequent were the stories of boys complaining at home about school beatings only to be beaten again on the basis that 'you must have done something to deserve it'. The traumatising of children was legitimised as the state 'condoned or ignored even blatant violations of the corporal punishment regulations'.[11]

The abuse he suffered in his school days left my father with a stammer and a reservoir of anger. He constructed fantasies of flight from the grey Ireland of the 1930s, learning short stories and poems, memorising by heart the poetry of the Romantics. Walking through the woods near his home, he recited Keats and Shelley until he cured himself of the speech impediment which the terrorising priest had inflicted on him. *Such a will*, I think to myself now, to create his own therapy for the trauma he experienced. He wrote and put on plays and went to the performances of travelling repertories who brought Shakespeare to the small towns of Ireland. The boy from north Kerry, a part of the country sneered at by urban sophisticates – its sons mocked as 'bogmen' – dreamed of being a famous actor. Through force of will and love of words he achieved an extraordinary transformation. By his early twenties he had been accepted into the Abbey Theatre school of acting. His career on the stage, screen and radio was launched. But already his drinking was registering as extreme, even in a society with a prodigious tolerance for the 'good man's fault'. No curtain call could cure that.

My father's alcoholism was rapid and self-obliterating. It was shameful to him, a skin he could not shed no matter how he tried – and he did, year after year, until it killed him at the age of sixty-four.

My father has been dead for over thirty years, yet still he comes, in the conscious hours of the day and in the night when I sleep. Sometimes he comes in a dream in which I am far out at sea, swimming to reach a boat. I see him below me in the murk, thrashing in the current and grasping for my arm to hold him. In this dream he is always on the edge of drowning. I do not reach for him. I swim to escape. I wake and my father has vanished again. I do not need a therapist to tell me it is a dream of loss.

Usually when I dream of my father, I am angry for several days afterwards. Or rather the dream releases the anger that is always bubbling. I isolate, because I know that I am not pleasant company. *Mr Angry lets you know with his vibrations from deep inside. Anyone in the room can feel them. Stay away, leave me be.*

The US Department of Veterans Affairs noticed a recurring theme of anger among patients in its hospitals. I flinched with uncomfortable recognition as I read their analysis: 'In people with PTSD, their response to extreme threat can become "stuck". This may lead to responding to all stress in survival mode. If you have PTSD, you may be more likely to react to any stress with "full activation". You may react as if your life or self were threatened.'[12]

Which was me. I was constantly stuck in the survival mode of PTSD. My response to any threat was to fight back twice as hard. A loved one said once: 'You act like the Ariel Sharon [Israeli leader] motto: "Always escalate."'

I am not physically violent, but rage has many expressions. I recall the precise moment of realisation. I was being treated for alcoholism and gritting my teeth through an interminable after-noon of group therapy at the rehabilitation unit. We drunks and junkies sat in a circle listening to each other's tales of shame. The therapists worked to break down our emotional protections. *But tell us what you feel, not what you think.*

'You're angry, aren't you?' one of the counsellors said, 'some-thing is making you angry.'

I was not about to acknowledge this in front of the rest of the group.

'No, I'm not.'

'You are. You've been angry all your life.'

I was being put on the spot. Up to now I had used evasive eloquence to protect myself from any forced revelations, an emotional politician deflecting and hedging.

As any good therapist knows, silence is one of the most power-ful tools they can deploy. The minutes passed. I felt the eyes of the group boring into me. I erupted.

'Fuck you. What do you know of my life?'

My expletive-fuelled fury lasted for several minutes. When I stopped there was silence.

We broke for coffee, and I went into the garden and sat under a tree and cried my heart out. The counsellor I had harangued walked over and sat beside me. 'I want to tell you a story,' he said. We sat there for the next hour and I listened.

His father had been a bully. He humiliated his son. His escape came when he was sent to boarding school, followed by army national service during the Cyprus Emergency. Afterwards he became a businessman, driven to prove he could succeed. His bank accounts filled up. He worked and partied hard and he became an alcoholic. Gradually but inexorably his inner torment rose to make a mockery of the public image of a high-rolling man about town. He went into rehab and got sober. When he came out, he sold his businesses and trained to become an addiction counsellor.

Despite all his years of therapy and helping others the ghost of his father still hovered. After his father's death he was given an urn containing the old man's ashes. But instead of putting it on a shelf, or even storing it in the garage of his large house, he took it into the garden and kicked it from one end to the other. 'I wanted to kick the old fucker all my life. I never got the chance. And now here I was, sober and in late middle age, walloping his ashes around the garden as if they were a football. I hated him.' That evening, when the river was in flood tide, he took the urn to the Thames and sent his father on his way into the swift-running current.

'And has your anger against him gone?' I asked.

'No, it has not,' he said. 'But he doesn't own my head anymore.'

It is over twenty years since I was in rehab. I have no violent urge against my father's ghost. But I am still an angry man. The ghost of childhood PTSD is still operating. And oh, how I have added to that deep well over the decades at the wars. In the Freudian formulation of depression, I always end up turning that anger towards myself. I wear myself down with it, until I break.

There are libraries of literature devoted to psychological problems of the children of alcoholics. I've sat through countless self-help meetings where the same patterns have been described – of childhood worlds without boundaries where adults acted, and children reacted. US psychotherapists Ivan Boszormenyi-Nagy and Geraldine Spark coined the phrase 'parentification' back in 1973. In families where one or more parent is emotionally absent, or out of control, children step forward to occupy the role of the adult. At its root, they said, was an intense loyalty to the struggling adults. Everything revolved around the addicted adult.

In the early 1980s researchers began to define specific characteristics of children who grew up in alcoholic homes. I share some of those I've read in the abundant literature on the subject. They are vivid to me and so central to who I became.

The children of alcoholics:

Have trouble figuring out what normality is.
Seek approval and submerge their own identity.
Are frightened by angry people.
Judge themselves without mercy.
Become addicted to excitement.
Become dependent personalities terrified of abandonment.
Learn to practise deceit in relationships instead of instinctive
honesty.

In her landmark book *Adult Children of Alcoholics*, the American psychotherapist Janet Woititz, herself married to an alcoholic, explained how childhood was distorted by parental addiction. 'Other people saw you as a child, unless they got close enough to that edge of sadness in your eyes or that worried look on your brow … whatever others saw and said, the fact remains that you didn't really feel like a child. You didn't even have a sense of what it's like to have a child's feelings.'[13]

For much of the first part of my childhood we lived at 1 Ashfield Park, Terenure, a red-brick Edwardian house with four bedrooms, built in 1903 when the electric tram extended its range ten miles to the south-west of Dublin city centre. The street was created in a style of muted gentility, fit for an age when the old cycles of repression and rebellion in Ireland seemed a thing of the distant past. Nobody then saw the end of empire in Ireland looming. The red bricks and little gardens spoke of consolidation. Ashfield Park was a fit home for the civil servants, accountants and the small businessmen of the Catholic middle classes. James Joyce was born five minutes away on Brighton Square. William Butler Yeats had lived a short walk up the road.

My world centred around Ashfield Park, the echo of my feet running along the little lane that led to the park at Eaton Square, or the garden at the back of the Milroys' house, the first places I was allowed to wander on my own and where I first experienced the sensation of physical escape from the troubles at home. There were other kids in our neighbourhood with alcoholic parents. I had a good friend, a red-haired boy with a wide moon face, who said his dad was like my dad. He didn't have to say how. It was understood. Once he stayed the night with us and wet the bed. He was ashamed of this. My mother said it was no problem at all. Years later, when drugs gangs began importing heroin into Dublin, my childhood friend died with a needle in his arm.

Those years in Terenure have a quality of permanence in my memory unlike any other place that I have lived. There were times of reprieve: when, in good humour and sober, my father was a storyteller and a joker. He introduced me to the Marx Brothers, the Three Stooges, and I can still see his head thrown back in uproarious laughter at the surreal humour on the screen. In the days of calm, we might buy nets from bald Mr Cobb in the hardware store and go to fish in Bushy Park. But always the tightrope. Always waiting for a fall, walking past pubs and the fumes of porter and whiskey and close-pressed bodies, and fearing my father would be pulled in, in front of my eyes, in front of the whole street.

The dominant feeling of those years was anxiety. I became aware of my body trembling. As I grew older my nerves developed a life of their own. My face began to twitch. It would start with the eyes, rapidly blinking, and then spread to my left cheek, and in my teens to my neck – a riot of involuntary motion that was quickly noticed by my peers. It could invite mockery and bullying in the classrooms and playgrounds of my primary days. Sometimes I fought back. But I never won a fight. The twitching has stayed with me down all my years.

I learned to look for the slightest change in mood in those around me. I anticipated anger and sadness. In the language of PTSD, I was becoming a 'hyper-vigilant' child. I did not imagine then how useful these mental distortions would become on the front line of war reporting, or how painful in the world of love and family.

I knew when to vanish, how to placate, how to escape into my head or up the lane to Eaton Square, how to prepare a face that could give the appearance of happiness even if by now I had absorbed the belief that, in the words of Thomas Hardy, 'happiness was but the occasional episode in a general drama of pain'.[14] I became overly attached to my mother. On those rare occasions when I was separated from her, I felt an overpowering anxiety. I have a memory of a Sunday afternoon in the late sixties when two first cousins came from Kerry to visit. My mother decided to take them to the zoo but for some reason she left me behind. It may well have been a matter of cost. When she broke this news to me, I was bewildered. I could not understand what was happening. Most eight-year-olds might have sulked or even stormed off to their rooms, but I became hysterical. I recall running after her car as she pulled away down the street, the mortified faces of my cousins looking out of the back window. Had anybody been able to heed it, the hysteria of my reaction would have been a warning that all was not well in my young head.

Every childhood departure was an abandonment foretold. Later in my boyhood, I joined the Boy Scouts and went on a fortnight's camp by the coast in County Sligo. Some of the other boys came from tougher parts of town and I feared them. They called me a 'Mammy's Boy' because I called my mother from a phone box and asked her to take me home. It was said that if you were 'queer' they painted your balls black with boot polish, though I didn't know what the boys meant by 'queer'. I roamed off on my own across the dunes, my feet sinking into the soft sand between the marram grass, dodging the crisp, tiny, bleached skeletons of rabbits. How wonderful was the safety of those open spaces by the ocean, the freedom from fear, the sense of loneliness receding in the face of the wind. All my life I would feel this liberation beside seashores.

Goodbye meant forever when I boarded those trains of the holidays, my mother on the platform at Heuston station waving us off, and me swallowing my grief station by station, south across the Curragh of Kildare and the Bog of Allen, the endless midlands from Portlaoise to Templemore to Limerick Junction to Mallow, and then the long tunnel into Cork, a last enveloping dark before my grandmother's face loomed, warm and welcoming, out of the waiting crowds at Connolly Station, and only then the panic subsiding. Was this reaction extreme? Of course. But it told the story of where fear had taken my mind.

I am not a good prospect for confronting the challenges of Irish school life in the 1960s. By the age of twelve I have attended four different primary schools in Dublin and a fifth in Cork. Physical violence is still common in the Irish classroom.

When I first arrive in class at a Gaelic-speaking school in south Dublin, I am taught by a woman who seems to loathe the children in her care. She wears a dark suit, glasses and has short greying hair. On the wall behind her there is a cross of St Brigid and a portrait of the leaders of the 1916 Rising. I try to shrink so that she will not see me. My instinct for danger is correct: as the first week goes by, I see children smacked with a stick on their hands, or they are kept in their place with sarcastic comments.

Later I move to St Mary's College in Rathmines, a private school run by priests and famous for nurturing some of the country's most famous rugby stars. Maybe had I been a more psychologically robust child I might have stayed on there, found a way to fit into the rhythm of physical punishment that shadowed the place, but the pattern is set. I am constantly scared, alert to the sense of threat, the roar of an angry teacher, the swing of a cane.

There is something else. I do not experience it here, but it will come to define the worst of clerical power and immunity in the Ireland of those days. There are a few priests at St Mary's who prey on boys, but only decades later will they be exposed. One is Father Henry Moloney – the so-called 'Dean of Discipline' – who is also the rugby coach. In the court case years afterwards, a Garda says the priest 'would assault the boys in the corridors, classroom and in a storage room. He would put his hands down their trousers and rub their backsides and thighs.'[15] One of the victims says that after the abuse he had difficulty with drink and drugs and that he had turned to crime. He said he was 'successful but things kept "falling apart"'.[16]

Move on to a winter's morning and it is still dark outside, and we are in the waiting room of Terenure College. This is another private school. I think my mother believed her children would be spared the worst of Irish school violence by saving up to send us to fee-paying schools. It is true that middle-class parents might choose – if they were so minded – to challenge arbitrary brutality in a private school. The poor had no such protections. There was no alternative but to send their children to the schools run by the Christian Brothers and other religious groups. If the children failed to turn up because they were frightened of the brutality, or they came from broken homes where education was far down the list of priorities, or because nobody cared enough or was available to see that they turned up, then the police could become involved, and in this way a child might start down the road to the hell of the industrial schools where perverts in clerical robes could do what they wanted with you.

My mother is talking to Father Hegarty. 'Hego', as the boys call him, is broad and beaming and welcoming. I like him. He is sure everything will go well. I listen and hope that the priests and the boys will be nice here. There is a wooden table covered with a sheet of glass. It fascinates me. I can still see it and feel how cold it is to the touch. Winter is everywhere that morning.

I make friends at Terenure, the first real friends of my life. I like the funny kids, the joke-makers, the ones who hang back from the schoolyard scrapping and macho-posturing. They read books, make smart remarks, and seem, in their own way, to be free of fear. I want to be like them. There are some nice teachers here who encourage an early love of history. But there are still beatings. They use the cane and the leather strap. When I witness the violence inflicted on others it makes me feel sick.

Eventually I am beaten. It comes to us all, sooner or later. I remember the stinging shock in my palms, and the shame and the holding in the tears because you did not want your classmates to see you break. They call them 'biffs', the blows to the hand. The number six returns to me. The teacher's phrase – echoed by boys – is 'six of the best'. Of the best? Yes, the best. The best violence an adult is capable of bringing down on the open palm of a child.

God, the perversity of it. You can close your eyes to what is happening at the top of the class, but the slash and crack of it is still there. And the whimpering after.

The head of senior school is nicknamed 'the Cow' because he has a big nose. I see him sweeping through the grounds, his soutane swirling, his head pushed forward. He uses a stick that is weighted with pieces of metal to maximise the pain he can inflict. Long after I've left, John Boyne, who later becomes a bestselling novelist, is beaten so badly by the Cow that he is off school for two weeks.* 'It was a culture of beatings and violence,' Boyne remembers. 'It didn't take anything to trigger the teachers. They were tortured souls. Angry, bitter men who looked at the thirty teenage boys every day who had independent minds and their whole lives in front of them and felt nothing but resentment towards them. They wanted to hurt them because of that.'[17]

There were some paedophiles at Terenure too, preying on the children in their care. John Boyne was one of their victims. The abuse would go on into the 1980s. English teacher John McClean went to jail in 2021 for molesting twenty-three students back in the 1970s. Another was a priest from County Cork called Father Aidan O'Donovan. 'How is Mammy Fergal?' he would ask me. *Mammy.* There was a lisping creepiness to the way he spoke the word. O'Donovan coached rugby and produced plays. He would make boys sit on his lap while he molested them. A past pupil described O'Donovan's modus operandi: 'Apart from the sadistic beatings many of us endured, they were always touching you up and grabbing you. Fr O'Donovan was a well-known "kiddy-fiddler". I remember him putting his hand down the front of my

---

* John Boyne's novel *A History of Loneliness* is based in part on his experiences at Terenure College.

trousers and holding me while I was going to the toilet. That was the sort of twisted thing we were put through.'[18]

O'Donovan flickers from charm to evil as if a switch is being tripped on and off. I learn to navigate around him very carefully, to avoid his attention. My PTSD is helping me here, making me careful. Once we are backstage at a play rehearsal and a boy makes a mistake, something small that I cannot now remember. Suddenly O'Donovan is screaming and belts the boy across the face. It was Synge's play *The Shadow of the Glen*, and I had a small role. My parents were in the audience on the first night. But I could not find any words when my part came around. I stared silent into the hall. Afterwards O'Donovan shunned me. I think I was in a more protected position than many. My father was a public figure. My mother was a teacher and notably articulate. My capacity for spotting danger helped me avoid this loathsome man.

There was anxiety at home and at school. I went to class exhausted and struggled to concentrate. My stress symptoms intensified. My mother took me to the family doctor in Harold's Cross. There was not much we had to say to each other – I being eight years old and near demented with fright, and Dr Oulton a stooped, lugubrious figure speaking beyond me to my mother. Was I getting enough sleep? he posited. *But wasn't that why I was there? I was getting no sleep.*

Later my mother took me to see a doctor in Rathmines known as Jimmy 'The Pill'. He prescribed sedatives. Years later he was struck off the medical register for his liberal dispensing of tablets. The medication deadened my night terrors. Had I been given a psychological assessment with today's scientific knowledge I am convinced that I would have been diagnosed with post-traumatic stress disorder.

The story of childhood PTSD is the story of life with my father and a society still in hock to clerical power. But it is not until later in my life, in the middle of my adult battles with PTSD, that I start to wonder about the trauma that came before my father, the story of what happened to his people, and those who went before them, my small farmer ancestors from the edge of the country.

3

Generations Fighting

Our ancestors live on in us as we'll live on in our descendants,
it's not that they live metaphorically in our volatile memories,
I thought, they live physically in our flesh and blood and our
bones, we inherit their molecules and with their molecules we
inherit everything they were, whether we like it nor, despise it
or not, accept it or not, whether we take it on or not, we are
our ancestors as we will be our descendants …

Lord of All the Dead, Javier Cercas[1]

It was the early summer of 1994 and I had driven from Uganda
into a vast graveyard. White butterflies swept in clouds across the
road. The rancid, offal reek of the dead rose from pits, ditches,
houses, the banks of streams and rivers; a smell that settled in the
mind as much as it lingered on our clothes and turned our stomachs. We came to a municipal building which was being used as a
temporary orphanage. The Tutsi rebels had rescued several dozen
children who had been hiding in the bush outside the town of
Byumba. Their parents had all been hacked or clubbed to death.
Several of the children had terrible wounds to the head and upper
body, inflicted by spears, machetes, clubs. There were some volun-

teer nurses who sat and spoke with the children. They spoke softly, in the hushed voices of the void after massacre. I noticed that we were being observed from a distance by a solitary little girl with a bandaged head. She sat and rocked back and forth. The girl was around four years old and had not spoken since she was found by the Tutsi soldiers. What a sight we must have been. Perhaps they had seen white men before, the UN peacekeepers who could not prevent the descent into butchery, or perhaps not. But our strangeness unleashed terror in her.

These children were not part of my familiar catalogue of intrusive memories and dreams, but they came back when I was researching the history of the Great Famine in County Kerry and asking whether what happened in those years might have left the imprint of trauma on my ancestors. A story of the long dead and what was seen in the years of the Great Hunger.

There is, in the account of an Irish land agent, William Steuart Trench, a description of unusual behaviour among children he encountered in the Kerry town of Kenmare during the Famine years of 1845–50.

Trench was crouched over his ledgers, noting rents received, those in arrears, the impossible cases who would never pay, those whose evictions were looming, when he heard a strange noise coming from the direction of the Kenmare workhouse. When he went out to investigate, he found that some children had barricaded themselves into a large room, 'mad with fright'. They believed there was a fire in the building. But the land agent could see no sign of it. When Trench forced open the door, he found the children 'fast losing their senses with terror. The eyes of some were already staring wide, almost idiotic in expression. Others had clenched their little fists, and ground their teeth, and threatened me in the most furious manner ... it was a dreadful scene of terror and despair, and the panic was evidently increasing.'[2]

Outside Trench saw eighteen to twenty children lying on the ground, 'some with their eyes staring and their bodies working in hideous contortions, some were completely idiotic from the fright. Some were quite motionless but doubled back as if under the influence of the cramp or tetanus. Some were apparently dead.'[3] What had happened? It appeared that one of the children had become convinced there was a fire, the fear had quickly spread through the entire group and created a collective terror.

These were children whose parents lay in mass graves in the surrounding countryside. They had witnessed horror piled on horror in the preceding months, as famine and disease killed thousands. Unmoored from home and family they were by now conditioned to expect fresh disasters. The workhouse itself was far from being a place of security. One in five of those who died in the Famine perished inside the walls of workhouses from hunger and disease. Nowadays the children Trench encountered would likely be diagnosed with PTSD.

But there would be no diagnosis, medication, or therapy for the traumatised children of the Famine. The acceptance of trauma as a psychic as well as physical wound would not appear until the end of the nineteenth century. It would take the cruelties of the Great War to lead to more enlightened evaluations of those previously dismissed as lunatics or cowards. It was still later – well into the twentieth century – before the concepts of epigenetic and inherited trauma became accepted fields of psychiatric study, as medical scholars began to investigate for how far into the past the lines of trauma might stretch.

* * *

Centuries of trauma hiding in plain sight. The first record of my paternal grandmother's family in the area dates to the 1820s, when they were tenant farmers in Lisselton, eight miles from the town of Listowel – and a mile or so from the Atlantic – where my cousins still work the land. Eight years before the Great Famine the *Topographical Dictionary of Ireland* described Lisselton as a 'parish composed of 6,327 acres of which only 300 are arable, 1,860 is coarse pasture the rest is bog and mountain'.[4] There was not much ground to yield food. Every acre was hard worked.

The Purtills farmed by a coast of harsh winter storms. They faced onto Tralee Bay and saw the ships heading to New York or Boston or Montreal, the escape route for hundreds of thousands. Long before the Famine my forebears existed as the chattels of chieftains and warlords, uprooted by war and the remorseless expansion of English conquest, exposed to relentless violence. Famine and killing laid waste to north Kerry in the sixteenth century.

They had the ruins of besieged castles and the collapsed cabins of the dispossessed to give a physical frame to their inherited stories of war and hunger.

My forebears did not look with hope on the world.

As a child my grandmother Hannah Purtill listened to the stories of the last Famine survivors. Her grandfather, John, was twenty-two when the catastrophe occurred; her grandmother Julia was the same age. There were uncles and aunts with vivid memories of those times. Her own father, Edmond, was born in 1850 and grew up in a land dotted with mass graves and empty cottages. Every boreen* in their home parish of Lisselton could summon its own platoons of the dead. There was no therapy for the trauma, but there were stories – stories told around the open

---

* From the Gaelic *bóithrín*, a laneway or small road.

fire in the pre-electric gloom of North Atlantic winters. The story-tellers spoke of the 'hungry grass' where those who died without the comfort of prayers were buried and which, it was said, left anybody who walked across it with an eternal, insatiable hunger.

A ghost story. A few years after the Famine, a man was walking home from Listowel to Lisselton. It was close to the end of harvest-time and he had gone to the town to take a drink with friends. But after a few bottles of stout and some songs he had an urge to go home. There was still more work to be done and he wanted to have a clear head when he went into the fields at dawn. As he passed the graveyard at Galey, where so many of the Famine dead were buried, he heard the noise of a football match inside.

There, he recognised neighbours he hadn't seen since the years before the hunger. How could this be real? he wondered. They were all long dead and gone. But there was warmth in the air, and they were full of joy to see him. The spirit of believing was on him. They welcomed him, shook his hand and invited him to join the game. As it happened, the Lisselton team was a man down and ten points behind. He jumped the wall and played the game of his life. When it was over, they sat amid the tombstones and passed around bottles of porter and spoke of times past. They enquired of him about people who had left for America and about new tenants on the land they had once farmed. Were they decent people? Did they take care of the ground? He answered each man's enquiry as best he could. But after nearly an hour of close ques-tioning he became exasperated.

'Sure, can't ye go and look for yourselves and see?' he asked.

The heads around him shook. They could never go beyond the graveyard wall. *But when you come back and play with us next week maybe you could bring news of the parish?* Some had kin who had died in the time of the Famine but had yet to join them in the world of souls. They feared they might have gone to the dark place. *Will you ask after them? Bring us news please, please, for the love of God.*

Promising that he would, he got up to say farewell. At the wall of the graveyard the man who had acted as referee, an older man who had been a rambling poet in the district, caught up with him. 'I'll have you down to play full-forward next Sunday.'

The younger man was nervous now and made his excuses. 'Well, I will if I can, but you know how busy it is in these harvest times.'

With that he vaulted back over the wall and made his way home as the first light was appearing in the sky over the Atlantic.

Within the week he had fallen dead in the fields. My father told me that story. Someone else further back had told it to him. A psychologist might describe this as the mediation of trauma through storytelling. The Purtills and the Keanes of that time lived in a world without therapy, without doctors to diagnose disorders and to listen to the emotionally wounded; how else was the immensity of what had happened to be expressed?

The Famine dead were people who had farmed beside the Purtills, who had played football and drank with them afterwards, who hunted the wren on St Stephen's Day, and danced around bonfires on May Eve and who, in the dark months of 1847, starved to death and drained away into the earth with dysentery. They were not gone. They were all around.

It may be sufficient to say, that their grief was wild, disconsolate and hopeless … an oppressive agony of remorse such as no language can describe.

The Black Prophet, William Carleton (1846)[5]

The Purtills were survivors. The facts of why one peasant family survived and another perished are unfindable. And even if the facts could be discovered, if it could be known that my people lived because they were lucky to have stored some small feed, or were physically stronger and able to work, or better able to fight their way to the front of a queue, or were just lucky or tougher or a combination of some or all of these things, would it change history or make the past morally comprehensible? It would not. We were not there. We did not live with the penance of survival – the 'moral injury' that is twin of post-traumatic stress disorder.

In the fields where the dying was done, there was only the imperative of survival, to do what had to be done to emerge alive.

I read the history. I try to construct a vision of those years as my people knew them. *What did they see, those Purtill men and women trudging back and forth in those lonely fields on the edge of*

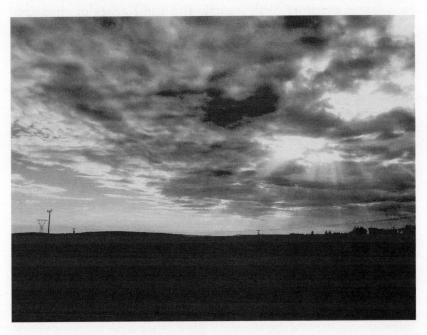

Atlantic fields at Lisselton, homeland of the Purtills.

the country? In the aftermath of the Famine, and well into my lifetime, a silence surrounded the question of survival. A sign on a mass grave near Lisselton declared '*An mbás siud a thug beatha duinn*' ('It was their death which gave us life'). But the truth we could not face was that they were not lives freely given. There was no sanctified martyrdom. The strongest survived; the weakest were obliterated. The burden of horror was never equally borne. Depending on where you sat – in the peasant's hovel, the land-lord's mansion, the strong Catholic farmer's house, the city tenement – the Famine affected your life in different ways, or hardly at all.

At the height of it a farmer told a visiting observer to Kerry that 'they died, as the birds do when the frost comes, and what we thought we never would see: they were buried without coffins'.[6]

What we thought we never would see. This is the story I would later know, the story of all trauma: the mind struggling to accept the evidence of the eyes. *Did it really happen? Did I imagine the whole thing?*

One year into the Famine the parish priest in Lisselton reported an increase of 500 per cent in the number of deaths compared to the previous year. Dogs followed the carts hoping a corpse would fall off. They too were ravenous. The historian Bryan MacMahon has described how at the end of a day ferrying bodies to the death pits, one of the drivers would go to the edge of the ocean and walk his cart into the sea, the waves washing away the stench of his lost neighbours.

The poet, and future President of an Irish Free State, Douglas Hyde, spoke of the survivors, with Darwinian enthusiasm, as 'men and women of the toughest fibre. They have been for gener-ations fighting with the sea, fighting with the weather, fighting with the mountains. They are indeed the survival of the fittest.'[7] This was romanticised nonsense from a man who hadn't known a day's hunger in his life. But he was right about survival of the fittest.

Community solidarity often collapsed under the pressure of hunger. Those suspected of stealing food could be brutally treated: a destitute woman was beaten to death in County Tipperary for taking a few sheaves of corn. Famines are, wrote one historian, 'always and everywhere, deeply *divisive* tragedies. The charity and solidarity that bind communities together break as the crisis worsens.'[8] This is a large part of the trauma of the famines I have known.

When folklorists went into the Irish countryside nearly a century later, they unearthed numerous stories of humanity breaking under the stress of hunger. In Rathmore, forty miles south of Lisselton, a man told the story of a woman he found trying to drown her daughter in a well. When he tried to stop her, she is said to have replied: 'Oh sir ... if the Lord would only call on her I'd be all right. Isn't it better for one to be gone than to have we all gone. She has a wonderful appetite and nothing could give her enough ... I must do away with her altogether or she'll starve the rest of us.'[9]

The stories collected from the oral tradition are not an official history, nor can they always be proved. But they speak loudly to the people's preoccupations. The dying, the exile, the trauma of witness, the degradation, the shame of not being able to save the ones you loved or those who lived beside you.

They looked back once,
Black moons of misery,
Sickling their eye-sockets
A thousand years of history
In their pockets.

'A Farewell to English', Michael Hartnett[10]

When it began, Ireland had a population of eight million, with 1,600 people in 'lunatic asylums'. Sixty years later, the population of the country had been halved and there were 17,000 in asylums. By 1914, the Irish Inspectors of Lunatics would conclude that an 'exceptional' number of asylum-dwellers were born during the Famine years, and that 'children born and partially reared amidst the horrors of the Famine and the epidemics of disease that followed it were so handicapped in their nervous equipment as to be weak-minded from the start or to fall victims to mental disease later'.[11]

Many of those committed to Irish asylums were older people abandoned by families who had emigrated, or who were thrown off the family farm after it was inherited by an older sibling. Others were simply the rural poor for whom the asylum was a better bet than roadside destitution. Still it appears – as one some-times sceptical scholar puts it – 'reasonable to conclude that the Great Irish Famine ... increased the risk of mental disorder among persons who were in gestation during the Famine and born during it or shortly afterwards'.[12]

My great-grandfather, Edmund Purtill, Hannah's father, was conceived in 1849, at the height of the tragedy. His mother, Julia, gave birth to three children in the Famine period, at a time when fertility rates were dropping dramatically across the affected areas of the country.

The trauma of the Famine changed my people. It gave them a Holy Trinity of obsessions. They worried for the ground beneath them. Land – the owning, holding, and consolidating of it – was their great preoccupation, and woe betide the man who tried to take it away, or strayed uninvited onto their fields.

They wanted things that would last. If there was no land to inherit the alternative was to study and join the civil service, or become a teacher, or enter a religious order. I had aunts and uncles who did all of these. My grandmother was obsessed with education: we should shine and get good degrees. The world was a stage on which her kin had to achieve, to become a somebody, not a nobody who could be swept away by history's next disaster.

The abundance of disease in those years helped bequeath an enduring terror of illness, particularly in rural Ireland. There are few families who won't recall a relative who suffered from recurring mystery pains and illnesses, and the fear of an early and painful death caused by cancer.

It has frequently been averred by politicians, priests and Irish humanitarians that the reason the country gives so generously to disaster appeals is because of the experience of the Famine. As the Irish Department of Foreign Affairs puts it: 'Ireland's own experience of hunger during the Great Famine in the 1840s still resonates today.'[13]

I believe the deepest impact of the Famine in my family came through political violence, the end to which inherited memory drove them. When the call went out to rebel against British rule in 1916, stories of 'the Great Hunger' were re-told, with much justification, as narratives of British callousness. As one historian acquaintance put it to me, the violent Revolution in the early twentieth century was 'a cry of revenge for the Famine'.[14]

On hearing that cry, my grandmother, who had lived among Famine survivors, joined the struggle. In her idealistic youth, she could not have seen that the war for national liberation would raise new ghosts.

4

Her Wars

'Our bad time is in front of us,' I said, and overwhelmed by
some vague terror, I broke down and cried. Women do not cry
much in Ireland during this war: the trouble goes too deep.

Kate O'Callaghan, Cumann na mBan[1]

I was not the first of my family to break down, or to know the
terror of war. Hannah Purtill was fifteen when the Revolution
began. By the time the fighting stopped, seven years later, she had
been changed by what she witnessed on country lanes and on the
streets of Listowel.

War in north Kerry would become … the broken corpses of
comrades after torture, the blood of a policeman congealing in a
gutter, the revolver pointed towards the head in a threat of execution, and night after night waiting for a battering on the door.

She is around seventeen years old when she joins Cumann na
mBan.* The leaders of the failed Rising have been shot, thousands

---

* The women's paramilitary organisation – the Women's Council – founded in
1914 that worked alongside the Irish Volunteers and later the Irish Republican
Army (IRA) during the Irish Revolution of 1916–23.

are arrested, and Lloyd George is threatening conscription to feed the war machine on the Western Front. Much of the country is enraged. Older pain surges to the surface. The executed rebel leader, Patrick Pearse, had harked back to the Famine when he urged the Irish people to rise up, calling starvation part of 'a profound polity'.[2] By 1918 militant nationalists in north Kerry were mobilising for war. There was excitement, the stuff that floods through young people when they have never known killing. What my people called the 'Tan War' began the following year. Hannah Purtill did not want to be a handmaiden who made sandwiches, prepared bandages and darned socks for the guerrillas, not when her older brother Mick was already ambushing policemen and British soldiers.

Hannah becomes a spy. This has costs. To be active is to risk your life and expose your family and community to British reprisals. It also means taking part in killings. The targets are often Irish policemen, with wives and children and who live in the community. It sometimes involves ostracising police families in shops, at social events, even at Mass.

It is a war of stalking, assassination, and reprisal. A guerrilla like Hannah might note a police officer's movements to and from the police barracks, establish their routine – whether they keep to the same hours every day, or stop at a particular shop in the morning or on the way home – and then take this information to the young men to plan an ambush, which means the gunman walking up behind a man and putting several bullets into his head and upper body before escaping, often handing the weapon to a woman who will take it to a hiding place. The departure and numbers of patrols are noted. Civilians making visits to the barracks are identified and reported to the IRA. Dealing out violent death is the objective. Suffering it is the occupational hazard. A bullet in the thick of the action, the hangman's rope in a city jail, torture and summary execution by a roadside.

As well as spying Hannah smuggles weapons and messages through military and police checkpoints. A lot of the women do this. But it takes strong nerves. At the time it seems like Hannah has strong nerves. The family joke was that she'd hidden guns in her knickers to avoid detection by the police. But as a child I did not make the connection between this levity and the facts of violent death on the village streets, or country laneways I knew so well.

I walk down Church Street today and into the Square. I stand outside the old Protestant church in the middle and try hard to picture sandbags around the Listowel Arms hotel to my right, and the military checkpoint on the bridge across the River Feale directly ahead, and police on the corner in their dark green uniforms watching who comes and goes. Anyone can walk up with a gun at any time and open fire. My grandmother sees all this as she goes about the business of spying. She has learned to deny certain feelings: until a few years before her family would have chatted amicably to the local RIC Sergeant and his constables. They met coming out of Mass and on fair days. She went to school and possibly played with his children. That would be unthinkable now. The RIC are all potential targets, unless they have secretly signed up with the IRA and are fighting the war from the inside.

I don't have a record of when Hannah first encountered the reality of killing, but I am guessing it is when they shoot Sergeant Francis McKenna in May 1920. He is thirty-nine and a father of three and a shotgun is discharged in his face. Two of his comrades are wounded. Hannah's good friend, May Ahern, hides the weapons after the ambush; Mick Purtill is possibly one of the gunmen as it is his unit and the shooting takes place near Lisselton. The women find hiding places for men on the run. They smuggle a wounded IRA man into the local hospital, where sympathetic nuns treat his wounds and keep him safe from search parties.

The government deploys two new units recruited from men who fought on the Western Front.* The 'Black and Tans' come from the ranks. The Auxiliary Police are made up of ex-officers. Reprisals become government policy, justified by Lloyd George in a speech in October 1920 when he says that '… in Ireland a harmless-looking citizen might pass a policeman in the street, and there was nothing to indicate that he had murderous weapons or to arouse suspicion. When he had passed the policeman he would pull out a revolver and shoot him in the back …'[3]

Heading into the winter of 1920/21 an atmosphere of terror envelopes north Kerry. The guerrillas attack a police patrol; a village is raided and burned in retaliation. Prisoners are tied to the front of lorries as human shields to forestall ambush. Others are dragged behind vehicles along country roads, leaving them battered to a pulp. One is tied to a horse and dragged across the countryside. Savage beatings of anybody suspected of IRA allegiances are routine. Many in the ranks of the Black and Tans and the Auxiliaries are already brutalised by years of horror on the Western Front.

The feminist and nationalist campaigner Hanna Sheehy-Skeffington is an eyewitness to the terror. She knows from personal experience the consequence of what can happen when a mentally unstable soldier runs amok. Her husband, Francis Sheehy-Skeffington, was murdered in 1916 by an officer from

---

* The strength of the RIC was more than doubled during the war by the addition of 13,732 new members, the majority of these 'Black and Tans' and Auxiliaries. The name Black and Tans derived from the mix of military and police uniform worn by many due to the shortage of regular police uniforms.

Cork, Captain John Bowen-Colthurst, who was badly traumatised during the Great War having already fought in South Africa
and India. He is a case study in war trauma. An inquiry after the
retreat from Le Cateau in 1914 found that he was 'in a condition
of marked nervous exhaustion and was quite unequal to any
strain, stress or excitement, which would probably bring about a
nervous breakdown'.[4] They sent him to Ireland with tragic consequences.

Women who transgress – in the eyes of the fighting men, or
their communities – are brutalised. Both sides shave the heads of
women they suspect of consorting with the enemy. The Black and
Tans have a reputation for sexual violence. Women 'knew not to
approach the Black and Tans as they were known to "molest and
mistreat" girls round the back of the barrack in Listowel'.[5] They
were notorious for drunkenness. Alcohol and trauma intersect in
the violence they inflict on others and, occasionally, on themselves. One Tan takes his own life in a pub in Listowel, while
drinking with fellow officers. Charles Ingledew from Inverness
has stayed on in Listowel – despite being discharged – for reasons
that are not clear. Perhaps the Great War veteran cannot leave the
new war that has become his home.

People are fingered by IRA intelligence as spies, then abducted
and shot dead, their bodies left on the roadside with signs
proclaiming: 'Spies Beware of the IRA'. Two police are kidnapped
in north Kerry and tortured. They are released but five weeks later
one suffers a mental breakdown and cuts his throat. There are
bodies bleeding out on the street, bodies buried in bogs where they
will never be found, lying from one century to the next deep in the
peat; there are bodies that are still alive being beaten and kicked in
the cells of the police barracks or, like the young trainee priest
home on leave for Christmas, battered to death in the town square.

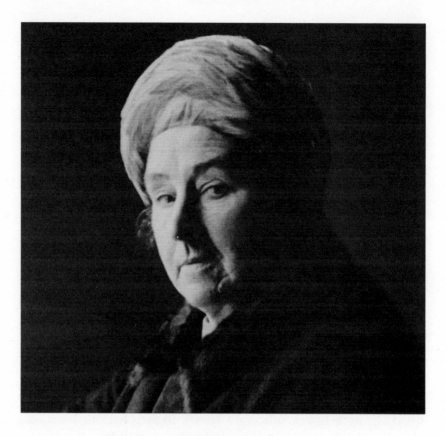

Hannah, my grandmother and war veteran.

The IRA shoots District Inspector Tobias O'Sullivan of the RIC. He is a father of three young children. He lives a few minutes up the street from the Keane family home on Church Street, where my grandmother would go to visit her future in-laws. His wife Sarah sees the blood flowing from his ruined head. She dies within a year. Some say she is broken by grief. O'Sullivan's movements to and from the police barracks on Church Street have been tracked by spies. As one of the assassins remarks: 'We had been informed of his regular movements by a number of scouts in Listowel who had been put on his trail as soon as the order was received.'[6] It is as simple and irrevocable as that. In my grandmother's house he becomes a ghost story, a green figure who stalks the house after dark.

Four local IRA men walking along the road outside Listowel are picked up by the Tans, badly beaten and then lined up before a firing squad and shot. Despite being wounded, one runs for his life and survives to tell the tale. My grandmother, Hannah Purtill, is among the group of women detailed with making sure the dead men are given a decent burial in accordance with the rights of the Church, and the customs of the country. A Cumann na mBan member who witnesses the arrival of the bodies at Tralee barracks recalls that 'the face of one young fellow whom I knew personally was all smashed in'.[7]

A few women are given the job of tending the bodies and are verbally abused and beaten. They find the dead men dumped in a shed used by the police for storing turf. The women wash and clean them. How easy to write that, and then stopping myself and imagining these countrywomen painstakingly cleaning away the blood and gore and then bringing the dead men back to Listowel, where the Tans and army have surrounded the train station. There is a stand-off which the women eventually win. The corpses are allowed to be taken to be waked at home. My grandmother is ordered to get nameplates made for the coffins 'at great personal risk to herself', as one witness puts it.[8] The women smuggle the guns into the graveyard, encircled by Tans, so that a military salute can be fired by an honour guard over the grave of one of the dead, Jeremiah Lyons.

I am talking about a small place here. All told the population of the town and its large rural hinterland is around twenty thousand people at this time. When something bad happens there's no hiding the details. Someone will always know someone else who saw it or was close by. This is how trauma gets shared around in time of war. Every violent act begets consequences that fly out into the community. There is not only the fear of the physical revenge that it might provoke – who might be singled out to pay the butcher's debt – but the grief which is both immediate and endless, and the way people start to lose trust in each other as they are unmoored from the certainties of the world of order that they knew. Sometimes a nastiness appears in people who were good neighbours before it began. When a retired local policeman, James Kane, is killed by the IRA as a suspected informer, his family is boycotted. They are refused service in shops and forced to walk long distances because no taxi will take them. The brass nameplate is removed from their front door. They live among people who wish to erase their presence.

In the British National Archives I read the letters of Kane's traumatised children and feel shame at the hatred that engulfed some in our town. James's daughter Elizabeth was, like my grandmother, a draper's assistant in Listowel. After the killing 'the staff refused to work with her' despite her having been an employee for fifteen years. She could not find another job.[9] 'After our father's death,' Elizabeth wrote, 'people whom we looked on as our friends turned their back on us and at one particular social entertainment (the first I attended in the town after our father's death) I was the only girl ignored.'[10]

A younger sister had a nervous breakdown and became 'a complete wreck'. The adult Kane children became destitute and were evicted from their home in the centre of town. In the years that followed a brother was murdered, robbed and thrown off the bridge in Listowel; another, a wounded veteran of the Great War, left for England because of threats to his life. The family was scattered and vanished from the story of the area. The silence closed in. When Elizabeth's lawyers wrote to a local solicitor to try and gather evidence in support of her claim for compensation, they were told that 'there is a great reluctance to admit having taken part in a boycott of this kind, or on the part of anybody to give evidence against neighbours … all parties in Ireland are anxious to forget the troubles of the years 1921, 1922 and banish them as a hideous nightmare'.[11]

There is no study of the trauma experienced by Revolutionary combatants and civilians in the seven years that began with the 1916 rebellion and ended with the last shots of the Civil War. The Revolutionary army did not have a medical corps, much less specialist psychiatrists who could diagnose or treat mental wounds.

In file after file in Ireland's military archives there are references to 'nerves' or a 'collapse' or 'nervous breakdown' or 'neurasthenia'. As early as the 1916 rebellion, hospitals were reporting civilians being admitted with 'melancholia' and 'mania' due to shock. The wife of Limerick's murdered Sinn Féin mayor noted in 1920 that 'owing to the tension due to outrages there was an abnormal number of patients suffering from nervous complaints and disorders'.[12] Outrage was a word that covered a multitude of frightening possibilities.

Often, I find myself stopping at a description whose symptoms I recognise. An IRA prisoner, on his release from military custody, gave an account that would have echoes for anyone suffering from war-related PTSD.

My nerves were completely gone. For the next eighteen
months I had the awful experience of being afraid, and it was
my first acquaintance with fear … At night, when asleep, if a
motor car stopped within hearing distance I would spring on
to the floor. All in all I had a rotten time.[13]

Trauma floats up repeatedly from the files. Like the report about the IRA men who were so affected by 'the strain [which] had affected their nerves' after killing eighteen Auxiliaries – veterans of the Western Front – in a Cork ambush that 'they were practically useless from that time on …'[14] This was the world of violence – sudden, ruthless, alien to her upbringing and instincts – in which my grandmother became enmeshed while still in her teens.

I am reading her military file when that line of Yeats, written in the middle of the war, comes back: '*The night can sweat with terror as before.*'[15] I read what she shared with doctors and the civil servants of the Department of Defence. By the time I am done reading I wonder how she could have avoided being traumatised by the war.

The file contains Hannah's appeal for a military pension from the state she helped bring into being. When she applies for the medal in 1967, Hannah is in her late sixties. Her husband is dead five years. The children have all left home. Money is short. She needs the veteran's special allowance. First, she must get a war service medal. This is proof of deeds done in the name of the Revolution. Once that is granted, she can apply for the allowance.

The state wants to know what she did in the war. Hannah knows – it lives with her. Her friends know – and a lot of people around the town who stayed out of the conflict, they know too. The Tans certainly knew enough to make Hannah a target.

She reached out for testimonials from her old comrades, some of whom had fought on the opposing side in the Civil War. Something of what they had shared as young comrades in the face of the Tan terror still bound these women. Now they came forward to testify. 'She was with me on many occasions,' wrote

May Ahern, 'acting on instructions from the Flying Column.'*[16] Another comrade, Mae Brennan, said that Hannah 'carried out numerous duties that were entrusted to her and was most relia-ble'.[17] There is a note too from Jack Ahern, who took part in the killing of Tobias O'Sullivan, describing my grandmother as 'an active member' of the movement.[18]

And then I see a name: Darcy. It is a name from family stories, a man who symbolised all we thought we knew of 'the Tan terror', the men in folk legend who were 'unleashed from England's jails'.

The Tan Darcy. I had always pictured him as an Englishman. It would take the detective work of a younger generation of Irish scholars to reveal the truth of Constable William Darcy, and of how the trauma of one war sent him to Listowel, to become entangled in the trauma of another.

In all my dreams, before my helpless sight,
He plunges at me, guttering, choking, drowning.

'Dulce et Decorum Est', Wilfred Owen[19]

I show Hannah's files to my friend Professor Linda Connolly. She is a sociologist who investigates the part played by women in a conflict that has for too long been seen through the prism of male experience. She is also the descendant of Revolutionary veterans. Her husband Andy Bielenberg is an historian of the Revolution and comes – on both sides – from German families that resisted

* Flying Columns were mobile units of the IRA during the War of Independence. Its members usually moved across country on foot or using bicycles that could be carried off road, striking at Crown Forces and then vanishing into the countryside.

Hitler. A grandfather was executed by the Nazis. They will help me make sense of the documents. Linda and Andy are people who understand at a deep level the pathways between war and trauma.

'It is only our generation, the third generation, who are able to ask and answer the questions about women's experience of that time,' Linda writes to me. 'For too long that experience has been hidden.'

Women in the ranks of the guerrilla army, or those who were the sisters and mothers of IRA volunteers, could be targeted by the police and military, but so too were women deemed 'loose' by the IRA or accused of fraternising with the Crown forces. The abuse did not end with the conclusion of the Tan war. Linda has uncovered the truth of Margaret Doherty, a thirty-two-year-old intelligence officer with Cumann na mBan who, five years after being gang-raped by three masked officers of the new National Army, died in a mental hospital, broken by trauma.

By the time I meet Linda I have already written a book about the war in north Kerry, much of it centred on the killings that took place in and around Listowel. Had I known what she and other colleagues were to discover about William Darcy, my grandmother's part in that narrative would have read differently. But the new information has a right of its own in my story of PTSD and war.

Darcy must have encountered my grandmother at a checkpoint or during a search. In any case she makes an impression on him. Hannah is a striking-looking woman with coal black hair and vibrant green eyes and a mischievous smile. She has a quick wit that strangers tend to remember. Darcy used to call in on her at Moran's draper shop on Market Street, where she worked as an assistant. 'Walk out with me,' he says to her. 'You are my maid of the mountains.' He stops her on the street and repeats the demand: 'Walk out with me.' But in the climate of the time his words are laced with menace. The Tans from Listowel barracks are notorious for their predatory behaviour towards women. Hannah refuses his advances.

Hannah informs the IRA of the constable's actions, most likely through her brother Mick who is in the hills of north Kerry with a Flying Column. She and her comrade May Ahern are told to track Darcy's movements. On an evening in April 1921, they trail him as he leaves the barracks, following him through Listowel, down Church Street and towards the Square. But Darcy is resourceful.

In her letter supporting Hannah's medal application May describes what happens next: 'We discovered him in the doorway of the Bank of Ireland hidden from view. (It was during curfew.) Suddenly he leaped out at us with a gun his hand and threatened us and ordered us out of town.'[20] Later Darcy went to the shop where Hannah worked and repeated the warning: she could either leave town or be shot. Death and torture are all about. Yet she does not go.

Darcy continues to be a marked man and later that year he is shot and wounded. So the family story goes. He leaves Listowel for good, leaving behind a name that is only mentioned on those rare occasions the war is discussed.

But Linda and Andy discover that Darcy was not who I thought he was, not the dregs of an English jail but born to an Irish Catholic family in Lanarkshire, Scotland, where his father worked as a coalminer after emigrating from Donegal. At some point in the early years of the twentieth century the Darcys moved back to Ireland, and it was from there that young William answered the call of King and Country. In 1915, he enlisted in the Royal Engineers as a sapper with one of the 'Special Brigades'. These were the units that fired poison gas to asphyxiate the enemy and carried flamethrowers to burn men alive in the German trenches. They saw extremes of human suffering: poisoned soldiers foaming at the mouth, vomiting green bile, tearing at their burning eyes, men screaming as they burned to death wrapped in flame. 'It was a disaster for the soldiers' minds and bodies,' writes historian Wolfgang U. Eckart. 'The fear of "gas" was paralysing, and the wounds caused by most of the poisonous substances were terrible', creating 'dread and long-lasting traumatisation'.[21] But it wasn't so much the harm it did to the body, wrote one officer, 'as the harm it did to the mind … this harmless-looking almost invisible stuff would lie for days on end lurking in low places waiting for the unwary. It was the Devil's breath.'[22]

William Darcy witnessed all this when he was just sixteen years old. Like thousands of others, he had lied about his age when enlisting. After the battle of the Somme, with public outrage growing over the casualty rates of so-called 'Teenage Tommies', the government recalled and discharged all underage boys from the ranks. Cut loose from the comradeship of the trenches, but with the horrors of the war fresh in his mind, Darcy drifted until war began in Ireland in 1919 and gave him a purpose again.

He immediately enlisted in the Black and Tans and was sent to north Kerry. Here he found himself in rural Ireland, among people who were nominally *his* people – at least in faith and shared culture – but who hated his uniform and would gladly kill him. William Darcy was twenty years old when he took up his duties in Listowel, a year older than my grandmother.

Knowing what he had endured in the Great War it becomes harder to see Darcy solely as the fearful creature recalled in family stories and described in my grandmother's medal file. He was certainly a dangerous young man, but he was probably also a traumatised one.

Ironically, at the time of his arrival in Ireland, hospitals in the major towns and cities were treating demobilised servicemen suffering from war trauma – or 'shell shock' and 'neurasthenia' in the descriptions of the time. More than a thousand soldiers and sailors were admitted. The prejudice that viewed the traumatised as shirking their duty, men to be isolated, given electric shock treatment, shamed, and even executed as cowards, was being challenged by military psychiatrists such as W. H. R. Rivers, who advocated a 'talking cure'. In essence the patients were offered a very early version of the treatments I would be given nearly a century later, built around confronting war memories in safe therapeutic environments. 'It is … one thing that those who are suffering from the shocks and strains of warfare should dwell continually on their war experience or be subjected to importunate inquiries,' wrote Rivers. 'It is quite another to attempt to banish such experience from their minds altogether.'[23]

At the Richmond Hospital in Dublin traumatised veterans were given hypnotherapy, taken on day trips to the countryside, outings to the theatre, and encouraged to speak of their experiences. In County Kerry, men were treated at the main psychiatric hospital, St Finan's in Killarney, where, the archives tell us, people like soldier 'EH', who was admitted with 'daily symptoms of mania, restlessness and poor sleep' spent a year recovering.[24] He was fortunate and was never readmitted, unlike soldier 'JR' who first came to the hospital in 1916 but was sent back in 1920, because he was at risk of harming himself or others. He 'was unable to tell simple factors such as if he was married or not. He complained of pain, nightmares and sensitivity to noises.'[25] The tormented man would spend the next twenty years in hospital, until he died there in 1943. After leaving Ireland William Darcy followed many of his Black and Tan comrades in joining the Palestine gendarmerie to confront the Arabs because, as the Secretary of State for the Colonies, Winston Churchill, wrote they combined 'a military efficiency … with a certain ruthlessness'.[26] After Palestine there is no record of William Darcy but it is thought he went to Canada where he enlisted in the army.

The nightmares of war are stubborn. They belong to the families of the victims and, more than we recognise, to the families of the perpetrators. I sat one evening by the River Feale with Seán Ahern, whose father Jack was a comrade of my grandmother and was one of those who wrote to the Department of Defence praising her war service. He had taken part in the killing of District Inspector O'Sullivan. Seán showed me a photograph of his father, with Hannah's brother – my grand-uncle Mick Purtill – and their IRA comrade and friend Con Brosnan, taken at a wedding sometime in the 1960s. There is, about each of them, the guerrilla fighter's hardness still, standing rigid and unsmiling, men with memories of killing, the stories that can only be recalled among themselves, to be hidden from wives and children and never allowed to disturb the myth of the good clean war for Irish freedom.

Yet already, by the sixties, these men are relics of an Ireland the young are leaving behind. The young are not interested in the detail of who did what to whom, or in the faces of the dead which still come unbidden to each of these men. It is known that Con Brosnan goes regularly into the church in Moyvane where he lives and prays for those he killed, and that he forbids children to have toy guns around the house. Nobody asks him why. Decades later his grandson, Conor, a doctor who frequently deals with victims of domestic trauma, thinks of Con's later years and how he was overtaken by drinking and depression, and suspects his grandfather was suffering from PTSD.

Seán Ahern grew up in a peaceful Ireland. When I ask about his father, Seán's eyes fill with tears. He struggles to accept that his kind, warm-hearted, hard-working father could have killed in cold blood. 'I mean how could you live with that? To walk up behind a man and shoot him in the back of the head in front of his wife and child?' The seventy-five-year-old son of a long-dead gunman carries the trauma of what his father had done over a hundred years before.

Hannah's service medal was granted in late 1967. To get her special allowance she had to supply evidence that she could no longer support herself financially. The Military Pensions Board asked for proof that she could not take up a job, and so sent her to see their doctor. The physician reported that Hannah Keane was 'very tensed and depressed' and was taking medication for depression and anxiety. He further recorded that she had been a patient at two psychiatric hospitals, in Tralee and Dublin, where she was treated for depression. The family doctor in Listowel confirmed that Hannah was incapable of 'self-support', and that she suffered from 'high blood pressure and neurasthenia'.[27]

These references to Hannah's diagnoses and treatments are from the 1960s, more than forty years after the violence of the Revolution ended. There are hints elsewhere, however – including a reference in a family history to my grandmother having a breakdown and being hospitalised in the 1950s. There is also a sentence in May Ahern's letter explaining Hannah's delayed application for wartime recognition: 'She would have applied before but for nervous disorders.'[28]

The diagnosis of 'neurasthenia' could be used in the military files to describe what we call post-traumatic stress disorder. 'Hannah is clearly naming neurasthenia as part of the outcome of her participation in the Revolution,' Linda Connolly tells me. 'It would have been very traumatic. Hannah herself is inscribing in the archive, in the state archive what happened to her. And she would have consented to the explicit naming of neurasthenia in that application, as being something that is part of her legacy of involvement in that period.'[29]

Into this I place my own sense of my grandmother's character. I knew her as a sensitive person, alert to the emotions of others. She had a sense of mischief and was a sociable woman who delighted in the company of her neighbours. When she was young and caught up in war it was her fearlessness that stood out. But for such a woman to be part of the process of killing, and to live with the threat of death herself must have been an immense psychological burden.

I could not imagine – not until now, in the grip of my own struggles – the cost of war for my lovely grandmother. There were the other burdens in her life that I have described. I do not attempt to ascribe everything to the war. But it was there always, and I can only wish that she had lived in times when mental illness did not carry the stigma of failure, and a patriarchal society did not dismiss the psychological troubles of women as 'hysteria' or inexplicable bouts of 'bad nerves'. I wished that she could have had the chance I have been given to know that the darkness could be challenged with a therapy that knew what it was looking to cure. Like so many thousands of Irish women, Hannah deserved better from the country she fought for. I feel, more than I ever could as a child, a deep compassion and kinship.

* * *

I am back to the beginning of the journey into my family history of hunger and war. Did any of it make me more predisposed to PTSD? Growing up I *felt* the presence of disturbance in my grandmother; I absorbed the ghost stories and the fragments of war stories. But all this was atmosphere. The science I read is tentative. The study of epigenetics – the transference of trauma through the genes – is still young. And I am not a scientist.

I go to see a medical man I trust, himself the descendant of people who experienced dislocation and war, and a former President of the Royal College of Psychiatry. Professor Simon Wessely is the child of parents who fled Nazi occupied Europe in 1939. His grandparents were murdered at Auschwitz and Terezin. Trauma has been a large part of his life's work. We first met when he asked me to talk about my experience of PTSD to an audience of doctors, a daunting prospect which only his warmth and empathy made bearable.

Besides my alcoholic parent and all that went with him, am I more predisposed to trauma because my great-grandparents were born during the Famine, and my grandmother was traumatised in a brutal war? Were there genetic changes rooted in the famine that made Hannah susceptible to trauma when she went to war? And were these handed on to me? There is simply no way of knowing, he says, without studying a representative sample group from the same area, with ancestors born in the same place and subjected to the same conditions.

'I can't do it on one person. And that's fool's gold. And anyone who says they can, is actually probably quite dangerous ... What I think is much easier to understand and, I think, is also the most powerful, is the influence of our background. And it's absolutely impossible for you to have grown up in the household that you did, with the interests that you have, for that not to have the same effect on you.'[30] As it evolves the science may expand the under-standing and treatment of some of us who have PTSD. But it cannot change who, and where, I am now. The professor is telling me I must look more into the culture, the stories, the influence of the adults around me as I grew up.

I absorbed the echoes of Hannah's war, and what she carried from all those who went before her. They would be part of who I became, the places I went.

5

Hero Child

And for the sake of his honour, Ferdia came at their call; for to him it was better to fall before the shafts of valour, of bravery, and of daring than by the stings of satire, of abuse, and of reproach.

The Book of Leinster[1]

Nobody forced me. To drive up the road from Ruwaished to Baghdad and see the coach all shot up, stained with blood, the glass sparkling beneath my feet, and all of us in that mad convoy of twenty and more vehicles wondering what might happen if the Allied jets and choppers overhead mistook us for Iraqi fighters, the way they had the people on the bus.

Nobody forced me to be there on the day in Kabuga, Rwanda when I lifted the broken door and saw the rotting soldier beneath it, blackened and shrunken, the photo album of his wedding lying open on the ground beside him. Or to walk through Bab El Oued in Algiers, when the Islamists would have killed any Westerner they caught, and our police bodyguards were a target themselves. Or to get into the car that morning in Goma, after praying for my life, and take the long road into the mountains

77

with a guide we did not know, along the tracks where militias routinely ambushed.

Nobody forced me to climb aboard the plane flying into the besieged Angolan city of Menongue and film the starving children Joao and Domingo, and later accept rice from the mayor because it was the only food to be found, or to feel that it was justice that I myself became sick with dysentery soon after getting home. Or made me go into the East Rand townships day after day and get caught up in gun battles. Or to count colleagues among the dead and go back into the world that killed them. Or drive on those mornings when steam was rising off the jungle roads, past the soldiers checking for mines, leaving safety behind to go into land contested by the Tamil Tigers and the Sri Lankan army.

Nobody forced me but myself. I could have been a reporter in politics or sport – I was at one point in my youth a rugby correspondent – or moved away from journalism altogether, become a teacher or a lawyer. There was a period in my early teens when I dreamed of being a marine biologist. Wasn't the experience of childhood enough to send me running from any possible trauma?

It was the opposite. The psychologist Meg Jay writes of children who become 'supernormal', developing exceptional survival skills through exposure to adversity. In a home where fear repeatedly hijacks the child's amygdala, the ability to read moods and threat levels is imperative. 'Most resilient children do not know about the amygdala and so they cannot explain their extraordinary non-verbal skills, or how they manage to stay alert all day, and sometimes even all night. They are as puzzled as anyone at their uncanny ability to know when something "ain't right", and to react automatically to cues that sometimes they do not even know they see.'[2]

The therapists call the skillsets I acquired in childhood 'maladaptive' behaviours. But I relied on these skills when pulling up to a roadblock in the South African townships, or during the civil wars in Liberia and Sierra Leone, where jittery teenagers with guns held the power of life and death. Unconsciously I read their body language, facial expressions, tone of voice, and responded accordingly. I worked to de-escalate hostile situations, to make sure I presented no obvious threat.

Childhood gave me the talent for reading danger. It also gave me the magic trick of seeming to be in one place, but being in another place, being another person, entirely: I could be a hero in my mind.

The bigger mood music changes in Ireland. I am conscious of eruptions one hundred miles to the north. What happens in Belfast and Derry is, in part, the unfinished business of the Revolution in which my grandmother fought. It becomes the morbid background of Irish life for thirty years, and it will offer me the opportunity to prove myself in a conflict zone.

In the summer of 1969 rioting broke out in Belfast and Derry and quickly evolved into a conflict that would kill thousands, maim tens of thousands more, and traumatise God knows how many. The Troubles in the north of Ireland began when I was eight years old and were still going when I became a journalist ten years later.

The year before it all blew up, I went north on a school trip. I was politically clueless apart from my family's Revolutionary legends, and aware that I had crossed into a place that looked and felt different to my southern home. My father explained before we left that the British occupied this part of Ireland and that they would someday be kicked out.

There was a customs hut on the border where the bus was waived through. (Decades later I would queue at the huge, fortified checkpoint outside Newry, where the young soldiers tensed at the possibility of an IRA attack.) On the other side they had a motorway, the first I had ever seen. Their fields were combed and neat. In Belfast we traipsed through bright sunlight, past the Portland stone of the City Hall and the giant cranes of the shipyard, returning across the Lagan to a modelling shop in the city centre where I looked for figurines of Napoleon's Grande Armée. Only many years later did I learn that I'd been conceived in a theatrical boarding house in north Belfast, while my parents were touring with a repertory group. The Troubles would eventually place the boarding house at 179 Duncairn Gardens and its kindly landlady, Mrs Burns, on the front line of the conflict. The street became part of the Belfast 'peacelines', where walls of concrete and steel (some as high as twenty-five feet) separated Protestant and Catholic areas.

On the way home we stopped on the coast near Rostrevor and searched for eels under the rocks of the foreshore. We moved without drama from one part of the island to the other. This was the last year that most of us would willingly cross the border, before the ambushes and the checkpoints, and before the names of places and people we had never heard of became part of our daily lexicon: Bogside, Falls, Shankill – along with B-Specials, internment, Provisional IRA, Official IRA, the UVF, Bloody Sunday, Ian Paisley.

In August 1969, hundreds of Catholic refugees fled south, hundreds more would follow. With each surge in violence they came – in '69, '70, '71 and '72, before the conflict coiled into a long, hateful attrition. The northerners were taken to camps as far south as County Cork, where a local reporter described 'the children and the mothers ... how shocked they looked'.[3]

Belfast was a few hours' drive from Terenure. It was all there for us children to see on the television news. The Taoiseach, Jack Lynch, said the government would not stand by while Catholics were being terrorised. Plans were made to send weapons north to defend Catholic areas and our soldiers were sent to the border. There were rumours that they'd be sent across into Derry, effectively an invasion of the north. What then? we wondered. A war with the British Army and the northern Protestants? It was frightening and thrilling. What would happen if it spread south, what would we do then?

My father and I would sometimes listen to the radio together. Between the comedy shows and the plays, the announcer spoke of shootings and bombings.

A part-time member of the Ulster Defence Regiment has been shot dead near Aughnacloy in County Tyrone ...

A Catholic man has been shot dead on the corner of the Antrim and Cliftonville Roads in north Belfast ...

'We'll have to be ready to fight if it comes south,' said my father.

'Like Pearse and Connolly!' I chimed.

'The very same.'

In our street games we played the Irish versus the English. I was always Pádraig Pearse. *God help our naivety*, I think now. I worshipped Pearse – Magnificent Pearse, racing towards the apocalypse in the General Post Office, who said the millions being butchered on the Western Front were warming 'the old heart of the earth with the red wine of the battlefields';[4] and James Connolly, already wounded when the English captured him, tied to a chair, facing a firing squad. Connolly and Pearse, the heroes I longed to be.

In his cups and out of them my father spoke of heroic sacrifice. He performed in a benefit concert for the dominant leftist faction of the IRA, before the murderous split in the organisation. In those days it was still possible for a man like my father, a man of impulse, to retain an attachment to romantic nationalism, especially if it was allied to the socialist ideals that were dear to both my parents' hearts.

It had seemed so much simpler in those early days of the conflict. Nearly fifty years had passed since artillery opened fire in Dublin city centre. The public world in which we lived was defined by dullness. For a short while we could still nurture myths of war: the gloried last stand in the burning building, the good clean fight, the blessed martyrs going smiling to death. The kind of war that never was and never will be. Around the corner in Terenure village my father would point at the spot where the IRA ambushed a British Army convoy in 1921. The soldiers were driving down the road singing 'I'm Forever Blowing Bubbles', when an IRA man stepped out to throw a bomb and shouted: 'We'll give you fucking bubbles.' The bombs and bullets ripped through the soldiers and 'the state of blood and gore of the lorries left little to the imagination'.[5]

As a youngster of course I did not hear the truths of war – of the killing of informers; the torture and executions in the Civil War, the crows feasting on flesh scattered on the trees of north Kerry, the soldier with his face blown off on the road outside Terenure College. Only as an adult did I realise that our history was a shallow grave, where the dead beckoned from beneath the topsoil.

I arrived at my first school, the Irish-speaking Scoil Bhríde (established to ensure 'the spirit of the Pearse brothers is never lost'),[6] when the country was celebrating the fiftieth anniversary of the 1916 rebellion. One of Pádraig Pearse's sisters came to visit. We

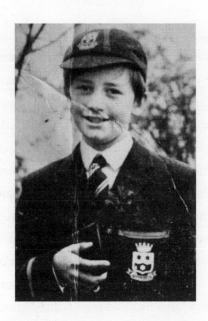

Dreaming of heroics. A schoolboy at the beginning of the 1970s.

marched around the schoolyard and sang a song of war written by her martyred brother: '*Óró, sé do bheatha bhaile*' – 'Oh-ro, welcome home'.

Sé do bheatha, a bhean ba léanmhar
do bé ár gcreach tú bheith i ngéibhinn
do dhúiche bhreá i seilbh meirleach
's tú díolta leis na Gallaibh

Hail, oh woman, who was so afflicted,
It was our ruin that you were in chains,
Your fine land in the possession of thieves ...
While you were sold to the foreigners![7]

Yet none of my schoolmates, to the best of my knowledge, were drawn into the ranks of the IRA, nor did any develop my obsession with war or self-sacrifice. Only it seems the melancholy boy on the edge of the playground, avoiding the games in which his peers knocked and shoved each other, was thinking of the days when he could show himself to be unafraid and have the world applaud him for it.

I was my becoming my own special case, the caretaker and rescuer of the adults around me, the 'hero child' trying to 'bring honour back to the family's image and identity ... disgraced by the presence of addiction'.[8]

War becomes flesh and blood when I am thirteen. Loyalist car bombs in Dublin and Monaghan kill thirty-three women, children and men, and injure hundreds more. I am safely in Cork, one hundred and sixty miles away, but the whole country is shaken. My friend John King is working in his father's business in Dublin city centre that day and the windows are blown in. He runs out to see what has happened. What he witnesses will send him into therapy thirty years later.*

Even in Cork, far from the northern war, we see troops protect banks and cash vans against IRA attacks. The police set up armed anti-terrorist units. A group of detectives become notorious for beating republican suspects, or what the government calls 'subversives'; the IRA robs banks and occasionally shoots police officers.

When he is drunk my father rails against the British. He wants the Irish Army to march north. But then the Provisional IRA starts

---

* There have been repeated allegations that British security forces colluded with the loyalist paramilitaries who carried out the attacks. An Irish government inquiry found that allegations of collusion made by a former member of the Royal Ulster Constabulary should be taken with 'the utmost seriousness'.

blowing people to pieces and shooting fathers in front of their children. Eamonn says his mother's generation would never have done such things. True, they didn't have 'no warning' car bombs, but the rest of it – the horrors children and wives saw when people were cut down in their hallways, sitting rooms, bedrooms, in their streets – they did such things, and endured such things at the hands of the state, and were mostly silent about them.

I know how messed up it looks now, but my childhood hunger to understand war began in that atmosphere. I fed it in libraries and through comic and magazine subscriptions. I read biographies of Bonaparte, Gustavus Adolphus of Sweden, Bismarck. I read war stories in the *Victor*, the *Hornet*, the *Hotspur*, where 'the Krauts' shouted '*Aargh!*' and 'the Japs' screamed '*Aieeee!*', as some plucky British Tommy dispatched them with bayonet or grenade. There were long evenings with my toy soldiers, flanking and encircling, painting Airfix models of ships and planes, and the excitement of opening parcels of lead figurines newly arrived from England.

On the few occasions my father and I went to the pictures it was nearly always to see war films. In 1966 he took me to the Classic Cinema in Terenure to see Walt Disney's *The Fighting Prince of Donegal*, perhaps the worst film about Ireland ever made, or even the worst film ever made, but I thrilled to the reckless bravery of its hero. We saw Rod Steiger as Napoleon in *Waterloo* and every British actor worth their name in *Battle of Britain* – that was shortly before the conflict up north quietened our cheers for the heroes flying Spitfires above the Kentish Weald.

A middle-class 'Mammy's Boy' who cried when he went away on a scouting trip was unlikely warrior material. But that did not prevent me from imagining glorious adventures in which I saved oppressed citizens in faraway lands, just as I sought to shield my mother from my father's anger. What formed in those years was the idea of war as a place where I could both banish fear and be praised: the affirmation of the crowd filling the void created by fear, fame raising the little boy above the shoulders of his tormentors.

My parents separated in 1972 and I moved to Cork city to live with my grandmother. The uprooting was traumatic. For the first two years my mother had to stay in Dublin, visiting at weekends. I missed her bitterly. On the day she went back to Dublin for the first time, I went on a school charity walk and was caught in a downpour and drenched. She had to leave before I returned. That night, for the first time in my life, I wet the bed. Every Sunday night after that, after she left for Dublin, I feared that she might never return.

I can see how the damage formed inside. It seems so obvious now, after decades of lived experience and therapy, how the brain gets messed up and protects itself with fantasies of escape, and hones the skills of manipulation and evasion. I sank deeper into my own interior world, into the libraries, the corners of school playgrounds, retreating further from a place where my facial tics and jumpiness, symptoms of dislocation and post-traumatic stress, attracted the bullies. I felt that I was strange – certainly unlovable – a feeling that has endured all my life.

Yet it is right to also call myself blessed. My maternal grandmother, May Hassett, kept faith in me. She was always there, always calm. She loved me unconditionally and made me laugh. Her house, covered in ivy and with a garden of apple trees and blackcurrant bushes, was an alternative model of home. Her husband, Paddy, also fought in the Revolution and never spoke of those days. He too carried a melancholy gene and suffered from depression towards the end of his life. But he died while I was still a baby, and I did not know him, except in the fond memories of his children.

As a teenager I began to come out of myself. A large part of that had to do with a change of school and the arrival in my life of a girlfriend whose welcoming family helped me to feel something more than strange. For a long while I found it hard to believe that I could be loved by a girl. Yet here was one who did so without hesitation. Only now, as I grow old, do I recognise this gift in all its importance. The school – Presentation Brothers College Cork – was run by a headmaster with a liberal outlook quite at variance with the prevailing ethos of the country. He encouraged me to learn about broadcasting and to write stories.* At 'Pres' I made good friends who, like me, felt increasingly alienated from the country around us. We despised the bleating of nationalist pieties while people were being butchered up north and occasionally in the south. I was a rebel with many causes. I joined the school debating club, arguing against political corruption, sexual conservatism, and the power of the Church – all the time dreaming of escape from the grey republic. I had also grown fond of the sound of my own voice, and the positive reactions of those listening to me in those draughty school halls of north Cork and County Limerick where schoolboy teams travelled to debate and flirt with convent girls.

Sometime in my mid-teens I decided I wanted to be a journalist. I could write reasonably well. I was interested in history,

* I have written before of my debt to Brother Jerome Kelly. He had been a missionary in the West Indies at the time of decolonisation and returned to Ireland full of idealism, and with a powerful sense of social justice. Words were not enough, he believed: righting wrongs demanded action. Much of my world view was shaped by this kind and brave man.

politics, and the world, and I came from a family with connections in theatre and the media. Both of my parents instilled in me a love of words. Nowadays my entry into newspapers – via a telephone call made by my uncle – would be scorned as nepotism. It was, but at the time all I could see was an escape route out and into the vivid world I was sure lay beyond the shores of Ireland. I had to start the journey closer to home.

I began my life as a reporter with the *Limerick Leader*, the main newspaper of the county from which it took its name, and learned my trade in courtrooms and at council meetings. But I hungered for foreign fields. In 1982, at the age of twenty-one, I persuaded the editor to send me to cover the Israeli invasion of Lebanon. Beirut was being devastated by air raids and artillery, hundreds had been killed in the Palestinian camps of Sabra and Shatila. It was the first big war in my time as a journalist and troops from Limerick were among the United Nations peacekeepers in the country's south. I got my inoculations, a visa to enter Syria – from where I would travel by taxi to Beirut – and some contacts for the Irish troops in southern Lebanon.

I knew nothing of war, knew nobody in Beirut, and had never travelled further than London. I was gormless and a danger to myself. A worried aunt got wind of the plan and contacted the editor, begging him not to send me: if anything happened, it would be on his conscience. He did what any sane person would do and cancelled the trip. I was bitterly disappointed. Gone was my chance of stunning Ireland with my courage and fine prose, of getting out of Limerick, and finding a world of wars. I needed a longer-term plan.

As a teenager I'd developed a passionate interest in South Africa. I'd read Alan Paton's novel *Cry, the Beloved Country*, Thomas Pakenham's history of the Boer War, the novels of André

Brink and the poetry of Breyten Breytenbach and Wally Serote. South Africa was the great moral cause of my younger days and I vowed that I would reach there before a race war tore the country apart. In retrospect, I see the projection that was going on. I would go to South Africa and face up to the bullies. Be brave. Be praised for being brave. I applied for a job in Cape Town, reaching out to a friend's friend on the *Cape Times*, but he wrote back to advise me that the apartheid state would not welcome a liberal white nuisance. Chances of a visa were nil.

I did not give up hope. I left Limerick for Dublin. I kept reading anything I could find about South Africa. I self-financed a trip at the beginning of the great township rebellion in 1984, my first experience of reporting undercover. In another two years I was back in the townships for Irish radio during the national state of emergency, nervously evading the apartheid security police. Five years after that I was the BBC correspondent covering the transition from racist autocracy to a non-racial democracy. I was an intensely driven young man, burning on those twin jet engines of insecurity and ambition. Nobody would have been able to stop me even if they wanted to.

In the lands between the Limpopo river and the Cape of Good Hope I would witness violence in a way that I had not in Northern Ireland. It was in front of me. So close that I had to step around it to avoid treading in the blood. I felt the pulse of 'war compulsion' in my veins – I learned that I was never more alive than in the presence of death. It would be close enough to kill men I knew. Perhaps me, if I was unlucky, or if I pushed my luck too far.

6

Reckonings

It may be he shall take my hand
And lead me into his dark land
And close my eyes and quench my breath ...

'I Have a Rendezvous with Death', Alan Seeger[1]

They were the ones with whom I roamed lawless lands. They were colleagues, competitors, comrades. They were brave, kind, crazy, selfish, stupid – some of the best people I have ever known, and some of the most broken: all pressed together by danger, excitement, curiosity, ambition, adrenaline, and things we could not then put a name to.

It is time to talk of those who did not come back from the days of killing in South Africa, and what they tell me of who I was becoming in those early days, when few of us had heard of post-traumatic stress disorder. Some were just unlucky. Some were brought to death by the seeds of pain planted long before, but that flowered in the madness of the conflict zone. They could have acted as my warning. Any one of their deaths might have persuaded me to stop there and then. Except none did.

I told myself that the precautions we took would keep disaster at bay. Death might caress as it passed by, but it would never embrace me. It was enough to follow the rules and I would be okay. Never drive down a silent road. Never drive down a road where people are fleeing in the other direction. Never race towards the sound of an explosion. Wear your flak jacket and helmet, even if there is no shooting at that moment. Most of the time that kind of knowledge, and a certain accumulated set of instincts about people and situations, in my case absorbed in childhood, kept war journalists alive. But in the places we went to in South Africa the rules had a way of changing very fast. There would be times when they failed us. And the longer you did the job, the more those times mounted up.

The first colleague I saw dying was Abdul Shariff, in South Africa on 9 January 1994. He was a talented photographer, and a sweet-natured man, thirty-one years old and careful about how he handled himself in the townships. This was more than a matter of attending to his physical safety. It could be measured too in his interactions with residents. He was respectful and he listened carefully. Abdul, a South African Indian, grew up under apartheid in the coastal province of Natal in a segregated neighbourhood. The man had real humility.

I remember the moment the shooting started. We were walking with a group of ANC leaders in Katlehong township to the east of Johannesburg. Nobody had expected trouble. The ANC delegation was there to hear from residents whose houses had been destroyed in factional violence. There would be the walkabout, the obligatory photos with the locals, and a press conference.

Then shots rang out. Everybody scrambled. I dived on the ground for cover. Single shots were followed by bursts of automatic fire. I did not dare lift my face from the grass on the roadside. When the shooting stopped I heard shouting. I leapt up and ran towards a group of four ANC fighters, carrying Abdul by his legs and arms. I heard him groaning as they passed. It was a low, exhausted sound, but I did not yet realise he was dying. I ran with the group to a car and remember worrying that their rough handling might cause even greater damage. The vehicle sped off, but Abdul was dead by the time he got to the local hospital. Poor gentle Abdul who just wanted to record what was happening to his country, who was no thrill-seeker or ego-tripper.

My colleagues and I took another wounded reporter in our car. She was lucky; the bullet had only grazed her stomach. A few centimetres the other way and it would have smashed around in her vital organs.

Two months later, on 9 March, my BBC colleague and friend John Harrison was killed in a car crash while we were reporting on fierce racial violence that had erupted in the north-west of the country. I went to identify and bring his body back to Johannesburg, a journey we made by helicopter because the roads were full of violent white extremists – the neo-Nazis of the Afrikaner Weerstandsbeweging (Afrikaner Resistance Movement) – who were attacking Black residents and journalists.

We collected John's body from the mortuary. All of it felt unreal. How was someone I had seen alive in the morning dead by the afternoon? I was wedged next to the body on the small helicopter as we flew home over the veld. A man I knew and respected, who had been generous to me, with whom I had some-times argued and oftentimes laughed, who in his life was a force of nature, a straight-talker for whom Mandela himself had a special affection, a loving husband and father of two boys, how was he now lying beside me wrapped in a sheet, strapped to a stretcher, and never to breathe again? Such were the times.

We mourned John and went back to work. His family scattered his ashes in the South African bush.

Nobody ever knew what the next day would bring, not the way we lived and the way the country was erupting. When Ken Oosterbroek of the *Johannesburg Star* went into Thokoza on 18 April 1994, ten days before South Africa's first non-racial elections, he already had four years' experience of working the townships. There was not much in the way of human brutality he had not photographed. Ken was one of a group of us who recorded the violence that accompanied the death throes of the South African apartheid state, but he was also part of a smaller band of photojournalists who were given the nickname 'The Bang-Bang Club' because of their reputation for close-up coverage of the fighting. I admired their courage and was grateful for their camaraderie. They respected others who regularly went into the townships to record what was happening. Like me they scorned the ones who pontificated from the safety of their offices.

We were predominantly male and in our late twenties or early thirties. Compared to those we were reporting on, we enjoyed lives of extraordinary privilege. Now, at a distance of nearly thirty years, I see how some of us were swept along by adrenaline and testosterone. Young men and war, the oldest story, where you learn, too slow, to never make bets on how it ends.

We blazed with righteousness. The apartheid state offered a clear target for all the outrage we could muster. Such a sense of purpose I felt. Like the day in June 1992 when President F. W. De Klerk arrived in the Boipatong squatter camp outside Johannesburg to sympathise with victims of a murderous Inkatha raid.* The fact that many of the ANC supporting residents believed he and his police were fomenting the violence and might not want him there hadn't registered with De Klerk or whoever was advising him. The visit descended into furious chaos. I crouched beside my car as the riot police opened fire on protestors with pump-action shotguns. Bodies went down. A man was killed. I phoned in live to the BBC in London but struggled to be heard.

I had no sense of fear at that moment. Only exultation at being there, in the thick of it, telling myself I was one of the chosen few, bearing witness for the world; and, when the shooting stopped, I felt the beautiful exhaustion that comes when the adrenaline rush recedes, and you know that once again you have come through unscathed. It was the same one day in Soweto when a shotgun pellet hit a man in the neck just a few yards away and he bled out and died because it had struck his carotid artery.

Some colleagues got hit that day. Minor wounds. We all got to go home to the suburbs and drink beer and feel good about our luck. Getting one over on the riot police by catching them in some act of awful brutality was our reward. Until eventually the risk morphed into a dead journalist lying on a township street, until the dead became people we knew, and the accumulation of hack and chop and bullets, blood and burning, and funeral after funeral, began to happen inside our heads even when it wasn't happening around us. What goes in must come out. Or go somewhere.

---

* Forty-five people were killed during the attack on the Boipatong informal settlement on 17 June 1992. The attack was carried out by supporters of the Zulu-dominated Inkatha Freedom Party, with the collusion of the police. The violence led to the collapse of negotiations between the African National Congress and the National Party government of President F. W. De Klerk and threatened to derail progress towards a non-racial democratic nation.

On the morning he was killed, Ken Oosterbroek was photographing a newly established peacekeeping force that was trying to separate the followers of the ANC and Inkatha.

The peacekeepers were a mix of men from both sides of the apartheid divide, mistrustful of each other, with vastly different levels of military experience.

When a gun battle erupted, Ken followed the rules. He took cover where he could, but the bullet found him anyway, entering his chest and causing massive internal damage. The bullets were flying in all directions that day in Thokoza. The coroner said later that nobody could be held responsible for his death. It is very rare for anybody to be held accountable for the death of a journalist in a conflict zone; there are usually more pressing priorities for the authorities. The more ruthless of them will sometimes be happy that the death of a journalist frightens others away from the scenes of their crimes.

Another of the Bang-Bang Club, Joao Silva, took a photograph of Ken, mouth open, life draining from his eyes, being cradled in the arms of his friend and fellow photographer, Gary Barnard. A friend of mine, Greg Marinovich, also a member of the club, was wounded that day, and later in different conflicts. He would eventually quit conflict photography, despite winning a Pulitzer Prize for his work. Greg had an insight, a sense of life's larger priorities, that took him off the road before it was too late.

Others of the Bang-Bang Club came to self-destructive ends. Kevin Carter took his own life three months later, on 27 July 1994. He was thirty-three when he died, just a month after receiving the Pulitzer Prize in New York. He should have been celebrating the prize and the new work opportunities that had come his way. But by the end he was gaunt and broken, chronically addicted to cocaine, and showing every sign of suffering from PTSD. In his suicide note, Kevin wrote: 'I am really sorry … the pain of life overrides the joy to the point that joy does not exist … I am depressed … without phone money or rent … money for child support … money for debts … money!!! I am haunted by the vivid memories of killings and corpses and anger and pain … of starving or wounded children, of trigger-happy madmen, often police, of killer executioners …' He ended by saying that he had 'gone to join Ken if I am that lucky'.[2]

Kevin won his Pulitzer for a photograph in Sudan of a starving small child who had fallen forward on her face trying to reach a humanitarian feeding station. A vulture watched the child from nearby. Along with the prize and fame came criticism and questions, the oldest question we face when reporting war: What had he done to help the child? Did he just leave her?

His explanation in his last days – and we are dealing here with a man close to collapse from depression, trauma and drugs – was that he had chased the vulture away, and the child had managed to get up and make her own way to the feeding station. I have met callous hacks whose only priority was the advancement of their own careers. Kevin Carter was not like that. He had the addict's curses of selfishness and manipulativeness, but he was a man deeply sensitive to the pain of others.

Kevin was not the only one to take his own life. Gary Barnard, who'd cradled the dying Ken Oosterbroek, never recovered from the death of his friend and mentor. Crack addiction took Gary to the point of no return. He eventually ended his life at home in Johannesburg on 13 September 1998.

Bad luck seemed to follow the group. Joao Silva, who'd taken the photo of Gary trying to help Ken, and of the wounded Greg Marinovich, kept going to the wars until he lost both legs in a landmine explosion in Afghanistan in 2010.

Archbishop Desmond Tutu was one of the first to publicly recognise the emotional cost of reporting conflict in South Africa in those days. 'And we know a little about the cost of being traumatised,' he wrote, 'that drove some to suicide, that, yes, these people were human beings operating under the most demanding of conditions.'[3] There was also something quite specific to their experience: they grew up in a society which traditionally prepared white males for colonial overlordship, funnelling them into compulsory military service – Carter had witnessed his first conflict as a national serviceman – and promoting a toxic cult of machismo. To the tender-hearted or the creative that country was a prison.

I knew these people and what had happened to them. My 'salvation' back then – if I can call it that – was that I didn't go down the route of hard drugs like Kevin or Gary. Alcohol was bad but it took me slowly. I have no reason to doubt, given my addictive nature, that crack would have quickly taken me to the end that killed my township colleagues. I was also, simply, one of the lucky journalists in the townships. There were moments when the bullets could have come my way, but they found other people, mostly Black South Africans – of whom 14,000 were killed in a conflict that lasted from 1990 to 1994.

I would like to give you the names of all the dead journalists I know – as colleagues, friends and acquaintances – for the memory of every one of them and what they sacrificed means much to me. But a list would be meaningless to you without also describing the life stories that are attached to each name. There are too many, and some of the mental pictures of their loss are too painful for me to retrieve and hold here.

Greg Marinovich described some of the feelings that came after the deaths of his friends in South Africa. He was brave in what he expressed about complex motivations and painful responses, the interweaving currents of guilt and loss, the reckonings with ourselves and our limitations that would eventually come home. 'At times, we felt like vultures,' he wrote. 'We had indeed trodden on corpses, metaphorically and literally, in making a living; but we had not killed any of these people. We had never killed anyone … Dealing with an intrinsic inability to help, our own inadequacy, is much more difficult, even impossible – we are always going to be inadequate to help all those who need it.'[4]

I questioned why I'd survived and others, who were more averse to risk did not. But most of the time I stored my feelings away: the grief for dead friends, the fear of being killed myself, the sense of failure for every situation I confronted where I felt helpless, the knowledge that the suffering of others was my daily bread, that I already knew this life was potentially fatal for me but that I would not, could not, stop doing it.

I was repeatedly re-traumatising, chasing a myth of who I wanted to be, exposing myself to violent people and places. But in those days of the early 1990s, I still had abundant energy to rebound from knocks and drive forward.

My hardest lessons of self, however, lay ahead, in a place that had been abandoned by the world. My adult life is divided between the before and after of that small country in the centre of Africa. It is my terra aeterna. I was not the same person after it, and I know that many others who were there felt the same. It left us with questions about humanity and ourselves that feel as if they will last a lifetime.

7

Believing

It's not been cathartic, more like digging up evil again and trying to put it into words ... Because there's an ugly side to this injury, not just a bad, stupid side, which is about the impacts it has on you. The ugly side is what the darkness does to the inner person and its significant impact on others.

General Roméo Dallaire, commander,
UN Assistance Mission for Rwanda, 1993–94[1]

I dread this part of the writing. Each time I return to it a thing happens in my chest, an acceleration of breathing which I know is a symptom of PTSD. A sweat starts on the back of my neck and runs down my arms and legs. The room is too small for what I am trying to set down. I want to close the laptop and go outside.

Sometimes I do that. I grab the dog and head for the fields. But not in the evenings, because there is a forest across the road from where I live and when the dusk shadows start to slip through the trees it makes me think of Rwanda. I see things sometimes when I walk down the pathways. Seen from a distance in fading light, a discarded coat crumpled up between trees can take me back to the place of the dead. If it's late in the day I just go to another room and switch on some music, or watch a comedy on my iPad, drink a cup of tea, and practise my breathing exercises. I fight the fear.

Tomorrow I meet Rizu. I must try to stop ruminating. I must try to sleep.

This is no ordinary encounter between old friends. Rizu arrives with an air of apprehension. The familiar energy is muted. For decades, whenever we've met, we talk about other things – family, work, the state of the country – everything except what happened when we set off down the road that led from the border on the Akanyaru river to the city of Butare in the summer of 1994, the experience we shared that lay in a past concealed by clouds and not to be approached, for only pain lay there and things that could not be altered.

Rizu has never spoken to colleagues about what happened back then, until now, after I phone her. Now the whole thing is back. But that isn't a bad thing – it has to be faced in the open some time, doesn't it? And it has come at a time when she is feeling stronger. In the nearly thirty years since Rwanda, she has fought other battles in life, raised children, lost a husband to cancer, seen her son come close to dying in hospital, left journalism behind, and embraced religious faith.

She says she can deal with what the past throws up.

Before we even start to speak of those days she looks at me and says: 'Stop beating yourself up. It's been long enough.'[2]

Rizu was the first to go into Butare. She went in on her own. It was Rizu who found us rooms at the only hotel still open, and then headed back to get us. When she thinks about it now, she asks herself: 'How the hell did I go in there alone?'

In those days we travelled without security minders. There were no risk assessments. Nobody said there would be counselling available when you came back. This was the world before the media bosses faced their responsibilities to those who went into the war zones. We simply found out what we could from colleagues and got on a plane. There were no mobile phones that worked in places like Rwanda. We did not have a satellite phone. Once we left the UN compound in Kigali there was no means of communication with base, or home.

It would have been impossible, Rizu agrees now, for anyone to have been able to describe to her in advance what it would be like. It is a common explanation among those who were there. The experience of witnessing genocide is not something that *can* easily be conveyed. She recalls another journalist trying to warn her before she left Nairobi – 'telling me, "You know you're gonna go and expose your soul to evil?" And I, kind of, brushed it aside. I said: "I have to do this."'

She wonders now if it was youth or stupidity, or the feeling that she had been given a job to do and simply had to do it. Rizu – Rizwana Hamid – spoke Swahili, having grown up in Tanzania. Her father ran several businesses there, before the family emigrated to Britain when she was in her early teens, a moment of climate and culture shock from which, she says, she never entirely recovered. I had already seen Rizu's sharp mind and physical courage on display in her reporting from the townships of South Africa, where we had first met.

Besides Rizu and I there were three others: the team leader and producer, David Harrison, was older than the rest of us by around thirty years – dogged and reserved in his emotions as seemed appropriate for a veteran officer of the Parachute Regiment. He had served in Suez during his national service in 1956; Glenn

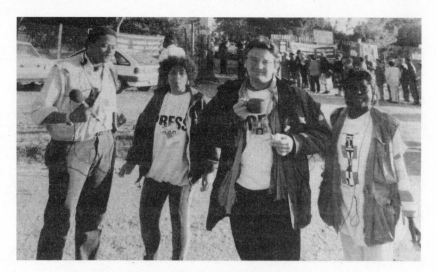

Rizu Hamid (second from left) in South Africa before we
left for Rwanda. (*M. Shipster*)

Middleton was the cameraman, born in what was then Rhodesia,
and who spent part of his youth in 'Boy's Town', a South African
settlement for troubled adolescents following the breakdown of
his parents' marriage; and Tony Wende, the sound-recordist,
another son of a 'broken home'. Tony was thoughtful, calm, witty,
the man who invariably stepped in to defuse tensions within the
group.

Before setting out from Nairobi it is decided that Rizu will try
to reach Butare, still under the control of the genocidal regime.
Some of the worst killing has taken place there and the
Interahamwe militia* are in the process of hunting down the
remaining Tutsis. She flies to Bujumbura in Burundi, neighbour-
ing Rwanda, hires a jeep, and drives towards the green hills.

---

* The Hutu extremist militia linked to the ruling MRND party and set up to
target Tutsis. The militia played a major role in the slaughter which led to the
deaths of as many as 800,000 people in Rwanda between April and July 1994.

Crossing the border, passing through one roadblock after another, Rizu sees the Interahamwe, their expressions of intense hatred. She sees fresh blood on people's hands and on machetes. She can smell the bodies putrefying in roadside ditches.

She finds a young army sergeant named Patrice who is friendly and offers to help bring the rest of our team through the roadblocks. Being a sergeant in the army in Butare, Patrice is possibly implicated in killing; the effort to exterminate the 'cockroaches' requires the participation of large numbers of military and militia. He might even be spying on us. But who cares if it makes our passage through the barriers easier? We accept his help in the spirit of necessity.

After finding accommodation at the only hotel still operating – the Hôtel Iluhiro – Rizu returns to the border to meet us. I write 'returns to the border' as if it were a simple matter of getting in a car and driving down a road. But once more she is forced to run the gauntlet of killers. We pass the same roadblocks days later. Most are commanded by young thugs with bloodshot eyes, high on weed and beer, dangling their grenades menacingly.

By now I have witnessed the aftermath of their work elsewhere in Rwanda. I have seen bodies piled in churches and in ditches and floating in rivers. I have listened to the accounts of survivors who hid under the rotting corpses of their families, to missionaries broken by what they have witnessed, to UN officers sick with despair over what they cannot stop.

To get to the border that leads to the city of the killers we have to come out of rebel-held Rwanda, and loop into Burundi – along roads where the Burundi security forces are busy prosecuting their own civil war – and then back into Rwanda and up the seventy kilometres of militia roadblocks to Butare. Throughout there is the constant possibility of ambush. We make brief crossings into the territory of the Interahamwe in Kigali and see more drunk, stoned, murderous sentinels, this time controlling access to the Red Cross hospital and the Hôtel des Mille Collines, where several hundred Tutsi have taken refuge. There is also the danger of being killed in shelling by either side as we traverse the valley between the Rwandan Patriotic Front (RPF) and government-held sectors of the city.* But in Kigali we have only to pass a handful of road-blocks to get to where we need to be, and are accompanied by UN peacekeepers. On the road to Butare our only company is the young Hutu sergeant.

Now that we are on the other side of the border, in the territory of the killers, I am full of fear. My stomach is in constant, swirling revolt. I struggle to drink a cup of tea without shaking. I am also angry and intolerant – what I recognise now as symptoms of extreme stress. I annoy Glenn with my sniping remarks about the lack of food and hot water, and make childish jokes at his expense. I think he wants to punch me. Who, for heaven's sake, complains about hot water in the middle of a genocide? I would have deserved that punch. Perhaps if I could have admitted my fear I might have been easier to be around. But I was determined not to show my anxiety.

Roadblock after roadblock. The killers search our cars for hidden Tutsis. They are also looking for Belgians, whom they blame for the oppression of the colonial past and accuse of siding with the RPF. At every checkpoint, Rizu keeps up an amiable patter; even when we are ordered out of our vehicles by drunken militia who demand 'gifts' before they will allow us to proceed –

* The RPF was the Tutsi-dominated rebel army that first attacked government forces in 1990 from its exile bases in Uganda. It subsequently signed a peace agreement but took up arms again when the genocide started.

Don't give them booze. Cigarettes okay, but no booze – she does not flinch.

But for every swaggering youth dressed in camouflage and carrying a machete there are many more who look fearful and abject. They ask if the rebel army is far away. Never again, they tell us, will they be slaves of the Tutsi. A more educated individual will come out from the crowd, a teacher or a civil servant unable to go to work because of the war, and offer themselves as a spokesperson for the group: they are fighting against an invasion; it is kill or be eliminated. Surely we can understand the right of a people to protect themselves? I ask my questions in the least provocative manner possible. The roadblocks are no place for grandstanding.

As we approach the city, we have no idea that nearly 300,000 people have already been murdered in and around Butare. Nor do we know that we are on our way to stay at a hotel owned by a woman who is directing genocide.

Butare, Rwanda's main academic and ecclesiastical centre, came late to the slaughter because, for a time, it had a brave Tutsi *préfet* (prefect), a government-appointed leader of the area, who spoke words of tolerance. Three-quarters of the city's population are Tutsi, a higher proportion than anywhere else in Rwanda, with a strong tradition of intermarriage with Hutus.

But, two weeks into the genocide, extremists killed the *préfet* and installed a man more willing to do their bidding. By the time the slaughter subsides, a hundred days later, in mid-July, Butare's killers will have accounted for approximately a third of all those murdered in the Rwandan genocide. Hundreds of thousands of Tutsis, citizens of Butare, and tens of thousands more who take refuge there, are hunted down, hacked, clubbed, shot, speared, set on fire, blown up – at roadblocks, in their homes, in forest and swamp, in churches, hospitals, outhouses, on the banks of rivers. This systematic slaughter is directed by a group of senior Hutu politicians, among them the Minister for Family and the Advancement of Women, Pauline Nyiramasuhuko, who also incites the rape of Tutsi women.

It is only years later I discover that in addition to being a government minister, Pauline Nyiramasuhuko is the owner of the Hôtel Iluhiro, a dreary, red-brick blockhouse on the road leading from the city to the border with Burundi, where for several days in June 1994, we stay as guests.

I notice that a member of the elite presidential guard – those who led the slaughter in Kigali – is on duty at the entrance to the hotel. But I put this down at the time to the family's exalted position in the country's academic life.

Pauline's husband is the rector of the National University of Rwanda, which lies to the south of the city. A quiet, bespectacled man who lives in the shadow of his more powerful wife, Maurice Ntahobari has a master's degree in mathematics from the University of Liège, and is always keen to pass the time of day if we meet in the hotel's gloomy corridors.

The couple's son is Arsène Shalom Ntahobali. Even in a period conspicuous for the elevation of sadistic killers, 'Shalom' – so named because he was born in Israel while his mother was on a government mission – will emerge as a notorious figure. Much of what he inflicts takes place close to his parents' hotel.

'In late April a roadblock was set up near Hôtel Iluhiro,' the International Criminal Tribunal for Rwanda (ICTR) finds.

[Shalom] Ntahobali manned this roadblock, which he
utilised, with the assistance of soldiers and members of the
Interahamwe, to abduct, rape and kill members of the Tutsi
population. The roadblock outside Hotel Iluhiro earned the
reputation of being one of the most terrifying roadblocks in
Butare, and the evidence established that it was the site of
numerous beatings, rapes, and killings of members of the
Tutsi ethnic group. In this regard. the Chamber has found
that Ntahobali personally raped and murdered a Tutsi girl
there ...[3]

If I stand in Rizu's room I can see a fire alight at the roadblock
just up the road from the hotel. Shadows catch the shapes of militiamen. Nobody passes through at this time of night, unless they
are soldiers or other militia patrolling the town. A Tutsi arriving
here would be killed straight away. Even a Hutu from out of town
could be in trouble. In the opening days of the genocide a
Congolese man and his wife, who happened to be driving
through, were killed in the market. The atmosphere is thick with
paranoia. Tutsi spies are everywhere, the militia say. Day and
night the hunt goes on for enemies.

Rizu goes to the forest to see a priest who has been hiding some
Tutsi. She is late returning, and curfew is minutes away. I watch
the shadows of the young men dance around the fire at the barrier.
Please return, Rizu. Come back safe. Come back now.

It is seconds from curfew when she gets back to the hotel. The
following day Rizu takes Glenn, the cameraman, with her to see
the priest. When they arrive he has changed his mind about
speaking to them. Somebody saw her outside the church previously and reported it to the militia. The Interahamwe visited and
asked him questions about the Asian woman. 'Glenn and I just

looked at each other, and we said: 'No, you know, we're not gonna push this guy. He's scared, he doesn't want to do it,' Rizu remembers. 'He was scared for his life.'[4]

She then tells me something that she could not speak of at the time. There is an image that sits with her, something she stumbled across when she was looking for a room in which to interview the priest. There were bodies near the church compound. She opened a door and saw a toilet. In the toilet was a rotting human head. Soon it would be just a skull. Tears are falling down her cheeks as she tells me this. Rizu has addressed this in therapy, but the grief remains.

The words run out. We sit in silence. I know better than to try and offer consolation. Sometimes when the past comes back it seems as if it was a story you were told, something witnessed by others. Other times it is perfectly real. For me there is no telling which version I will get.

As these horrific events unfolded throughout Butare and as the violence in other parts of Rwanda pushed people to seek refuge in places they considered safe like churches and government offices, numerous already traumatised, mainly Tutsi, civilians went to the Butare prefecture office seeking refuge. Hoping to find safety and security, they instead found themselves subject to abductions, rapes, and murder. The evidence presented by these survivors, and accepted by the Chamber, is among the worst encountered by this Chamber; it paints a clear picture of unfathomable depravity and sadism.

Judgement in the case of Pauline Nyiramasuhuko, ICTR[5]

We travel to the *préfecture* where we hear that several hundred Tutsis have gathered. They believe – or at the time I thought they believed – that they will be safer in this place, next to the office of Préfet Sylvain Nsabimana, the short, plump, softly spoken politician who had been installed in the job by the extremists because of his pliability. The refugees here are exhausted and fearful. The air smells of wood smoke and bodies long unwashed. I say to Nsabimana that I think these people will be dead by the time our film is broadcast in a couple of weeks. He replies that he does not think they will be killed. 'They have no guarantees, but they will not be killed,' he says. *No guarantees.* Our conversation is on video tape. I clearly suspect murder will be committed. It is a conviction that deepens when we go back to try and film the refugees at night and are turned away.

The criminal tribunal pieced together what had happened at the prefecture in the weeks before we came.

The evidence established that, around the end of April, the attacks started at the Butare prefecture office, when assailants began to abduct and kill civilians seeking shelter there. In mid-May, Nyiramasuhuko, Ntahobali, and about 10 Interahamwe drove to the Butare prefecture office in a pickup truck. Nyiramasuhuko identified Tutsis taking refuge there, and ordered the Interahamwe to force them onto the truck. Once full, Ntahobali ordered the Interahamwe to stop because the vehicle could not accept any more dead. The Tutsis were taken to other parts of Butare to be killed …

The Chamber has also found that on two occasions in the last half of May, Ntahobali and Interahamwe came to the Butare prefecture office. Ntahobali violently raped Witness TA, while the Interahamwe obeyed his orders and raped six other women. The second time Ntahobali ordered about seven Interahamwe to rape this same witness while he raped another woman. The evidence also proves that further attacks took place in the first half of June. During these attacks, Nyiramasuhuko ordered Interahamwe to rape Tutsi women, and Ntahobali aided and abetted the rape of Witness TA by seven Interahamwe.[6]

I had no idea at the time, either, of the sexual violence that was taking place; these crimes emerged later in the reporting of human rights groups and testimonies given by survivors at the tribunal. Protected Witness 'TA' told how Shalom Ntahobali had taken her behind the *préfet*'s office and raped her. A defence lawyer attempted to suggest that a woman filthy from lack of water to wash could not have been 'attractive' to the militia leader. 'Would you say that in the conditions you were in, not having taken a bath [Shalom interrupts], you smelt?'[7] This appalling crudity evoked gasps of astonishment in the courtroom.

This Shalom was the scion of the family that had housed and fed us. They invited us to watch television in their private quarters and cheered for the Republic of Ireland football team when we watched them play against Italy in the FIFA World Cup. They sold us beer and eggs and enquired daily of what we knew about the advance of the rebel army. All of this while Mrs Nyiramasuhuko and her son encouraged the extermination of the last Tutsi of Butare.

At the Hôtel Iluhiro, Pauline's husband introduces me to his deputy, the vice-rector of the University of Rwanda. The university has been closed since the start of the genocide. Most of its Tutsi students and academics have been butchered, although I am not aware of this at the time. The gardeners and janitors have vanished. The vegetation is advancing remorselessly after the rains.

The vice-rector is clearly a fanatic. I share some of a precious bottle of Irish whiskey with him: I need him to do an interview, so I indulge him with alcohol and small talk. His hatred of Tutsi people is quickly evident. Later, with camera rolling I ask:

'Do the Tutsi deserve what is happening to them?'

'Do the Hutu deserve what is happening to them?' he replies. 'War is terrible,' he says. 'People get killed.'

War is terrible. The stock rationalisation used since time immemorial. You tell the lies you need to tell in order to live with yourself, as the Israeli psychologist of trauma, Professor Gilad Hirschberger, writes: 'Perpetrator groups may deal with the dark chapter in their history by thoroughly denying the events, disowning them and refusing to take any responsibility for them.'[8]

'This is the nature of the world,' the vice-rector continues.[9] Whatever is happening to Tutsi civilians is an unavoidable by-product of the calamity which had been unleashed on Rwanda, not by him and his ilk, but by the Tutsi leaders of the RPF.

The vice-rector's calmly rationalised hatred and its day-to-day consequences penetrate my defences. I am angry. Not the anger that can come and go. The kind every human experiences. This is quite different. It has a quality of permanence that is not easily erased. Later I learn that the vice-rector was instrumental in inciting hatred against Tutsi students and fellow scholars at the university, and it is claimed he stood by while one of his senior colleagues was murdered at a roadblock.

My post-traumatic stress from Rwanda does not come solely from witnessing horrific scenes, or from the fear I sometimes felt for my life. What corrodes the spirit is to be in the presence of those who have been overtaken by a hatred so absolute it will not discriminate between combatant and civilian, man, woman, or child, those who are ready to excuse anything.

I will be angry at the killers for years, and unforgiving of myself, feeling that I had failed in Rwanda when confronted with the greatest challenge to my courage.

8

Abandoned

A feather carried her with it into a darkness
which no one could fathom …

'Farewell', Cheryl Ntakirutimana[1]

The chorus starts up before dawn with the deep-throated bellow-
ing of tree frogs and calling of birds, a music that would be
enchanting in a time of peace but which now fills me with fore-
boding. We are coming to the end of our time in Butare and
today face a journey through some of the worst checkpoints.

Every day has brought news of fresh rebel victories across
Rwanda. There is a growing panic in the city. *How close are the
enemy now? Will they do to us what we have done to them?* The RPF
is closing in on Butare.

From a hotel window I watch the militia stop a woman whose
bicycle is loaded high with her family's belongings – blankets,
clothes, pots and pans – and force her to unpack. They harangue
her but I cannot hear the words. She is eventually allowed to pass.
I can only assume that she is Hutu. No Tutsi would be mad
enough to try to pass, because even Hutus are being raped and
robbed.

I have no sleep. My sleeping pills are gone and the few beers we shared last night are not enough to bring on a drunken slumber. I leave the room and pace to the end of the corridor and back. I am impatient for the journey to begin. Once it has, I trust the adrenaline and some of those skills of survival formed in childhood to guide me down the path.

Leaving the hotel, I notice the presidential guardsman watching us with more than usual interest. He floats around our vehicles and equipment, saying nothing, but looking as if he is making mental notes.

There is a plan to evacuate several hundred Tutsi orphans across the border into Burundi. The evacuation has been organised by the Swiss relief organisation Terre des Hommes. Préfet Sylvain Nsabimana and a senior army officer are coming too. The *préfet* signs a pass allowing us to join the convoy. At the time I see Nsabimana as a lone voice of reason in the middle of the madness. Only years later, because of the evidence given in an African courtroom, will I discover there was more to this man than mercy.

We are told to arrive at the departure point at around seven in the morning. Through the night I have been worrying about the road between Butare and the border – about the killers who will see the trucks coming and wonder why they should spare the occupants who are, after all, the children of the 'cockroaches' they have been ordered to exterminate.

The orphans, who witnessed the murder of parents, siblings and other family members, have been living in tents pitched on a field around the Karubanda Social Sciences School. Nobody has studied here for months. For now it is a place of comparative safety – comparative in the sense that no child has yet been dragged out of there to be murdered, though four were taken from their previous refuge.

If the children can make it to the frontier they will be described as some of the 'lucky ones', those who have evaded the grand plan of genocide. But what luck is this that has murdered all they loved? The luck of one more sunrise but no guarantee of another. The luck of exile and a lifetime of nightmares. I have never before seen such fear as that reflected in the wide-open eyes that greeted mine when I looked inside the trucks that morning. Perhaps it was that being young, unlike the exhausted refugees at the prefecture, they still had some hope of survival. To hope in life meant you still feared death.

The girl who will help me years later is here. I have no idea of this. We do not know each other. She is hiding and I am too focused on all that is going on around me. She has been hidden for weeks. Now there is a chance she will escape. Later I will have lifelong reasons to thank her.

Up at the school they are almost ready to leave. A white man and woman and a group of Rwandans have been busy assembling the children and guiding them to the container trucks which will carry them to the border crossing at Akanyaru Haut, then on to Burundi to be collected by the Red Cross.

Some of the children are bandaged from attacks with machetes and clubs. On each child's clothing a number is pinned. In this way they can be identified by the volunteers who will greet them on the other side of the border.

We try to be discreet. Some of the children chatter nervously to try and hide their fear. The air is full of nervous energy. The white couple are Alexis Briquet, coordinator of Terre des Hommes, and his wife Deanna. They have already organised one convoy to the border, saving the lives of 400 children. There are some among the local extremists who see Alexis as an enemy. In May, he was approached in a bar and told by a university professor that the Swiss were known to have links with the RPF. He was subsequently arrested and thrown in jail before Nsabimana intervened and had him released.

To go to Butare on lifesaving missions takes extraordinary courage. There is nothing ostentatious about Alexis Briquet and he has no interest in self-publicity. Only people with the virtues of calm and exceptional patience can deal with the militia. He does not raise his voice or bluster; he has no army to back him up. He comes from a country that is neutral and with little global political power, certainly not in Africa, and his NGO is small with limited access to influential people in the UN. Yet, over the space of two months, his organisation has saved hundreds of children and some adults too.

The priority is to get the convoy moving early. Nobody wants to be on the road when darkness falls. Glenn and Tony travel in one of the trucks with the children. Rizu and I drive directly behind, and David behind us.

There are long periods of scared silence on the road to the border, and there are tensions that provoke arguments. Sometimes we have to speed up to keep pace with the lorry in front. I can see the young orphans' eyes staring from inside the containers, and I'm afraid that we will crash into them if we have to stop suddenly.

Rizu and I argue over the speed she is driving at. She says now: 'I remember you saying to me: "Slow down." I said: "I know how to drive." It was me saying, "I'm in control, I'm driving."'

I wonder now if Rizu wasn't also afraid – with good reason – of falling behind the rest of the convoy and finding ourselves alone with the Interahamwe.

At the roadblocks we show our passports to the militia and, as ever, Rizu shows them a relaxed demeanour when they ask to see our papers. *No, we are not Belgians. No, we have no weapons hidden. No, there isn't any beer in the car.* 'That is where the African side of me came out,' she says, 'because I would use banter in some places and be very humble and I'd exert myself as a woman in other places. I just kept thinking: *These kids' lives are in the hands of the convoy …* One thing positive that can happen in all of this is to get them to safety.'[2]

Each roadblock has its own personality, often defined by its current boss. Even though the road to the frontier is only thirty kilometres away, there are more than twenty barriers to pass through. One single belligerent militia commander could hold us up for hours. At some roadblocks they insist on inspecting the trucks and our vehicles. Every time that happens, we hold our breath. Militiamen holding clubs and machetes climb up and check inside, looking for teenagers or adults. On the last trip the children were held for two hours just outside Butare, even with the *préfet* and a military officer arguing their case.

At a place called Kigembe, the convoy is surrounded by an aggressive group of militia. Thousands have been slaughtered in Kigembe since the start of the genocide. The men on the barrier are all seasoned killers. The *préfet* and army officer get out and start negotiating with them. 'When you meet such people, you do not try to use force,' Nsabimana explained later. 'What was important for me was that we should leave the area safe and sound. There were no authorities there. The authority was the authority that was at the roadblock.'[3]

In between the barriers, Rizu and I speak of life and what we will do in the summer after leaving Rwanda and editing our film. I speak of my sister's upcoming wedding in Vancouver. After that I will spend some time in Ireland and then move on to Hong Kong to a new posting. Rizu will go back to Zimbabwe, where she is living, and try to start work on projects that have nothing to do with death and killing.

We reach the border post in the afternoon. There are soldiers milling around. The *préfet* speaks to their commander. Alexis Briquet moves back and forth between the orphans and the Rwandan soldiers and officials. This place saw terrible slaughter at the beginning of the genocide. The Italian consul in Rwanda, Pierantonio Costa, who accompanied the first evacuation of orphans, remembers seeing footprints on the ground where fleeing people had run through the blood of those cut down by soldiers and militia.

Looking at the footage of our arrival at the border now it is hard to sense the fear felt by the children. Television can only capture the most surface of emotions. It will frame a smile, a tear, a howl, but the obedience that accompanies true terror is beyond recording. What I see is a line of children – silent, compliant, the older ones holding the hands of the younger – walking across a frontier to safety and leaving behind the graves of those who had loved them, and the Tutsi refugees still trapped at the office of Préfet Nsabimana back in Butare. They become my echoing question.

I believe that by the time this programme is broadcast most of those people will be dead. They were my words to Nsabimana after seeing the refugees outside his office At the least, I had an acute foreboding.

Why did they not cry out to us for help? Fear, probably, resignation; after seeing so much death, were they simply waiting for what they knew to be inevitable? There were no peacekeepers to call upon. The militia was committed to their destruction and to that of anyone who assisted them. Or let me take the other troubling possibility, that in those few days they believed the gates of hell had been closed at last, and the appearance of international journalists suggested some normalisation? But why did we not say we would stay with them until help came, whenever that was, however long it took?

I talk about this with Rizu. She wants to be fair: 'I mean you guys had been through hell on the other side, in terms of that fear that at any moment you could die. There could [have] been an attack in the middle of the night, Interahamwe were everywhere. There were no guarantees. So, by the end of it, it was like, yeah, just "get it and get out".'⁴ You might also argue, as I am sure colleagues would, that our job was to get the story out to the world, not to shoulder the responsibility for those in world capitols who abandoned Rwanda in the first place.

All of this I accept to be true. But the question about leaving would live with me for many years.

The sense of helplessness took people in different ways. Rizu remembers a cameraman colleague who, after Rwanda, went on to cover war after war. But then he broke. He could no longer do what he was so brilliant at doing. He could not cope with the world anymore. So, he went to live alone on an Italian island. It would not work for me, I say. Rizu and I speak of what kept us going to places like Rwanda.

'You're on a roll and so you just do it,' she says. 'Part of it is adrenaline, part of it is ego, part of it's: "What's the next gig?", part of it is the pressure of it. But I think what that does to our soul – what it does to you as a human being – I think it's only when you stop that you actually understand.'⁵

Rizu reminds me of the moment in Nairobi, after we had returned from Rwanda and before going our separate ways, when we all sat down for a goodbye lunch. Beers were ordered and food.

Somebody started to cry. Then the rest of us. There was just silence and tears. Everybody then left the table and went to their rooms.

The aftermath took us all in different ways. Rizu stayed on in Africa. She suffered depression and went into therapy. Then came the death of her husband. Eventually she moved back to Britain.

Glenn stayed doing front-line news camera work for the BBC for another twenty years and then one day suddenly quit and became a wildlife photographer. When I had lunch with him in Johannesburg a few years later, I asked if Rwanda still came back to him. He nodded and said that in his dreams he heard machetes being sharpened.[6] He has suffered from PTSD.

Tony went to Afghanistan and across Africa as a news producer and magazine writer before he embraced his true gift and became a writer of fiction and children's books. Once in Nairobi, on another assignment, he said to me: 'It's believing it happened, that I was there, that I have trouble with.'[7] A therapist would say that the struggle to believe is the psyche's way of protecting itself against the horror.

Our team leader David, the ex-Para officer, put his emotions into his work, doggedly pursuing investigations about the causes of the genocide and the responsibilities of the great powers. Nobody would ever think he was emotionally scarred by Rwanda, but he could not let it go any more than I could.

Though I now realise that I suffered from PTSD long before 1994, Rwanda marked a turning point in my condition. I began to experience recurring nightmares and flashbacks. I resorted increasingly to sleeping tablets to get me through to the morning. I had so many questions. About how such cruelty can come out of the hearts of men and women. About me and my need for danger and about the borderlines of courage; and about the people we left behind and what might have happened to them. It never went away.

I drank more. I drank to forget. I drank from fear. Guilt. Shame. Anger. I drank because I was an alcoholic. Fear. Shame. Anger. Alcohol. My Four Horsemen of the Apocalypse, bearing me to a point of crisis.

9

Blackout Boy

All your life, the trail of ruin you leave.

'Deer Hit', Jon Loomis[1]

It worked for me. It worked like nothing else ever did or ever could. It was my go-to medicine for the symptoms of a disorder I knew I was carrying but to which I had yet to put a name. It kept working every year for twenty-five years, until it worked no longer.

The end came not in a crash but a slow sinking in a bar in northern Spain where a maudlin drunk sat staring into a glass that could not cure the riot of nausea in his stomach, the pounding in his head and the waves of pity – for himself, for those who loved him and those who had tried to help him. They call it rock bottom in the alcoholic world. I had heard enough testimonies from other drunks, in different parts of the world, in my long years trying to get sober. Some described horrific physical circumstances: waking up handcuffed in hospital and seeing two cops watching from the end of the bed; the woman revived for the umpteenth time after an alcoholic seizure only to hear a paramedic say: 'This is a fucking waste of time. Sooner or later this will kill her'; the man who pawned his brother's wedding suit on the day of his wedding to get money for a drink to stop his shaking; the woman who would hide behind a bus shelter, still drunk from the night before, to watch her two sons, whom she was forbidden from meeting, go through the school gates until one morning the youngest of the boys spotted her and started to cry and the older one put his arm around him and steered him away.

I believe alcoholism was always in me. It was there when I was born. Scientific research tells us that there is 'overwhelming evidence that genetic variations contribute to the risk for alcoholism'.[2] But it doesn't matter to me why I became an alcoholic. The 'why' doesn't change the facts.

I was around twenty-one years old when my drinking took me to the rooms of a doctor in Cork. He was a family GP with no formal psychiatric training. But he had enough experience of drunks to spot the problem quickly. He asked a few questions.

How much do you drink? Tell me the truth. There's no point in lying. I can't help you if you lie.

Not every day, but when I drink I get drunk.

When you don't drink are you thinking about drinking?

Yes.

And when you are drunk what are you like?

I start cheerful and end up really sad.

I told him about the blackout a few weeks before, when I passed out on a city street and woke up at the front door of my mother's house. Between the city and the house was a distance of several miles. I had no memory of what transpired on that journey.

There were other blackouts. After some I woke with my clothes soaking and muddied or carrying bruises where I had fallen or – I cannot be sure – been punched or kicked. Blackout erases time. It is a terrifying phenomenon. How to account for time when we are awake but not awake?

The blackout, and the deep melancholy which followed, were part of a pattern that had developed in the previous year. I was in my first job as a journalist and earning enough money to pay for drink, as well as availing of the abundant free booze at press receptions and parties. The atmosphere encouraged hard drinking. It was what people did, especially in the newspaper trade, and the scrapes people got into – blackouts, fights, car accidents, hospitalisations – were laughed off as a rite of passage.

Many journalist friends have rosy memories of their drinking escapades as young reporters. But it is not the camaraderie of late nights in the Railway Bar or Hanratty's Hotel, or the singing afternoons at 'Durty Nelly's' or pubs in remote corners of County Clare, that I remember, but frozen, hungover mornings on the platform at Limerick junction waiting for a train to the city, watching the wagons loaded with lumps of beet trundling south to Cork while my stomach heaved and dread drew in from every side; or the nervousness every time I walked the city streets that I might meet the bank manager who'd been calling me for weeks about an overdraft inflated by cheques written to publicans and off-licences; the memory of a night when in anger at myself I drove my fist through the plasterboard wall of a flat and, shame-faced, presented my wounded hand to a weary nurse at A&E. This by the age of twenty-one.

The doctor in Cork listened to half an hour of my truths and a few evasions and delivered his prognosis:

'This is not easy to hear at your age, but the truth is that you can never drink again. If you do it will kill you, eventually.'

I remember that his face displayed no sympathy. He wanted to frighten me into sanity.

I felt shock. It was less the prospect of forsaking alcohol than the explicit connection that had just been made with my father. I had the same disease.

I felt it first around the age of eight. There was a flagon of cider on the dining-room table. I remember the shape of the jug and the transparent glass through which I could see a honey-coloured liquid. My parents were celebrating Halloween. A turkey had been cooked. Such occasions were few, but I remember that they were both relaxed. As far as I can recall, my father was not drinking. I think my mother regarded cider as a 'light' drink she could drink in his presence. They were in the kitchen talking when I felt the urge to reach for the bottle. I tipped some of the liquid into a glass and swallowed. I felt my body warm and a delicious loosening of the nerves. Gone was the feeling of a body fighting against itself. I felt an otherworldly sense of relief.

And once I had taken that first drink it would wait patiently until I returned, however long it took.

I did not drink again until my early teens. Then it was an out-of-date bottle of Harp lager stolen from the drinks cabinet of my grandmother's house in Cork. It tasted vile, like I imagine fizzy drain water would taste, but I drank it furtively in a garden shed and again felt the warm wash of relief.

In bars from Belfast to Kinshasa and so many other conflict zones I chased that sense of relief, the one thing I knew would stop the constant sense of being under threat, and which would elevate a personality that was essentially ill at ease with itself, and others, into something that projected an amiable sociability.

As a teenager I discovered the pubs along the docks that would serve underage drinkers. They were the haunts of the down-and-outs and the overnight workers coming off their shifts. There was a weekend drinking cabal at school. On Monday mornings stories of drunkenness were traded in the schoolyard before class. We drank rum and blackcurrant, until one night I drank so much that I vomited my way home across the city. The smell of rum still makes me nauseous.

Even then there was a handful of boys whose antics suggested darker possibilities further up the road. One boy blacked out in the middle of lunchbreak and was taken to hospital by a sympathetic teacher, who came back afterwards and told us not to gossip about what had happened. He was later repeatedly hospitalised for alcoholism.

Another classmate became violent with alcohol and was arrested. When the whiskey had him, he attacked anybody – close friend or enemy.

I did not join the ranks of the obviously addicted back then. I dipped in and out of the heavy boozing scene, thanks largely to the influence of my girlfriend. It was she who arranged for me to see the doctor in Cork when I started to slide into tearful depression.

For several years I followed the advice of the Cork doctor. I did not drink. He prescribed anti-depressants, which I dutifully took although they made no difference to my mood that I could discern. I remember only that I was told not to eat cheese while taking them. The longer abstinence went on, the more I missed the drink. In those early days the idea of seeking help from other alcoholics through Alcoholics Anonymous was anathema to me. There was something shameful about going near such an organisation. I remembered that AA people came to our family home to try to fix my father. Their presence signalled to me that our misfortune was public knowledge.

After a couple of years of not drinking – as distinct from being sober – I inevitably found my way back to drinking. It started with a glass of champagne. A celebration of a new job. Who could begrudge a man a glass of champagne in his hour of triumph?

Pretty soon I was back to where I had left off.

I established a pattern that would go on for years. I would start by drinking as others drank. A couple of drinks with a meal, perhaps a couple more if we were at a party. There was nothing to outwardly suggest that I was in trouble. Usually that would last for a month or so. Then I would begin to drink away from the company of others, in pubs where I could be sure not to meet anybody I knew. Or I would stay up late on my own, going into the garden to open a bottle of wine or can of beer, away from the possibility that anybody might hear the cork unpopping or the ring being pulled on the can. There was a solution to that: place a blanket or a towel over the bottle or can to deaden the noise. Alcoholism is made up of endless deceptions, of others and most of all oneself.

I would stay out too late. I would fail to arrive at an appointment. I would make drunken calls from pubs with lame excuses, or blackout in the middle of telephone conversations. I would descend into morose silences. Sadness crept in and made itself at home. When I did not drink I thought of drink. When I drank I thought there would never be enough. I am still chastened when I think – as I must, for this is a disease of denial that never goes away – of the madness of sitting at a table and watching a bottle empty and wondering how I could justify ordering another, the incredulity of seeing someone drink a half glass of wine and not wanting more and me thinking they were the one with the problem.

Throughout my own descent, I was still trying to shepherd my father away from alcohol. I saw him through several rock bottoms, or what I thought were moments of truth in his battle. But they accumulated in his last decade of life, and every time he emerged from hospital, weaker and physically aged by the struggle, my faith that he had reached a conclusive turning point became harder to sustain, despite the sincerity of his promises. He really did wish to be well. But the power of his addiction was too great. It undid his own best efforts and the patience and kindness of those who wanted him to get better. To the end he was cared for and made welcome in the houses of friends and family. It was not enough. I think he understood, deep down, that alcohol would kill him. He certainly knew what it had cost him.

I believe that Eamonn loved me, but his ability to be a father in any meaningful sense was destroyed by addiction. He had been sober in the months leading up to his death. There was a small part in a Hollywood film of my uncle John B's powerful play about land hunger in Kerry, 'The Field', and he had a pension which was more than enough to meet his needs. By then he was living in Listowel. It was his hometown and there were plenty of family and friends who offered him love and support. Yet he drank again. By then he had suffered several heart attacks and doctors had warned him that death would follow if he picked up the booze again.

He was full of pain and the attempt to drown it killed him.

The funeral was in January, the middle of a hard winter – a world of bare trees, bogland, streams rushing with brown flood-water, a journey south along icy roads, across the mountains between Cork and Kerry, to a burial that was a public event in which I played my expected part. There were television cameras and newspaper reporters. I spoke at the grave and quoted the beautiful lines of F. Scott Fitzgerald, another victim of alcoholism, from the last pages of *The Great Gatsby*, in which the narrator recalls Jay Gatsby's 'extraordinary gift for hope, a romantic readiness such as I have never found in any other person and which it is not likely I shall ever find again'.[3]

This was true of my father. I can see something brave in his attempts to try again and again to beat alcoholism. This acknowledgement of his courage can coexist with anger, loss, fear, all the muddle of feelings which childhood left to me.

I did not cry. I was engaged in a performance. Looking back now I am embarrassed by myself. I was far removed from real feelings. But my father would have understood. In that sense I was his actor's apprentice: the poetic gesture by the graveside, the dignified restraint of the public mourner, the eldest son in the perfect pose of maturity. I did not know then what I felt about him. I was numb and dissociating. Whatever was happening was not happening to me. I left Listowel the same day as the funeral. I did not drink – it was during a sober interregnum – but I would again, soon enough. The numbness only departed years later when I was being treated for PTSD, and I could weep for the sorrow of family we lost and the life he might have had, the grandchildren he could have known; and I would weep for my own drinking and failings, the deficiency of courage which impelled me to avoid honest confrontation in everything but my work.

I understood the connection between Eamonn and me and booze, the bonds of history and genes that propelled us both to the bottle, but it was not enough to stop me. I lied. Again and again. I said I was not like him. My alcohol issue was different, I told myself. I could always get a grip and stop.

I drank in Belfast, Johannesburg, Angola, Cambodia, Congo, and everywhere I could along the road. The feeling of relief that came with the first glass never faded. But the hangovers and depressions got worse. I began to be afraid. I would step into the shower pledging that I would not drink that day. By the time I emerged my resolution was upended, and I was at the minibar throwing back the first whiskey of the day, sour and savage and soothing all at once.

In those days the life of a correspondent in a conflict zone was filled with opportunities for hard drinking. In my own mind I was part of a special breed of men and women who risked everything, high on my exceptionalism as an anointed warrior for truth. The trauma of war zones was real and relentless, but it also provided me with an alibi.

Who would not drink seeing the things we see?

Alcohol was the legitimate and time-honoured medication for the horrors we witnessed and the risks we took. This was the long decade when the wars of the former Yugoslavia, the horrors of Somalia and Rwanda, and the roller coaster of South Africa, forged a generation of journalists who believed they had looked into the eye of evil and found the courage to confront it and alert the world. Time would prove my naivety. I think often of Stephen Spender's poem 'The War God' and its rueful lines, 'for the world is the world ... and it writes no histories that end in love'.[4]

The same people met in the same places. Colleagues succumbed to the bottle and to drugs. Marriage after marriage fell by the wayside. There was fierce competition, but also a shared contempt for those we saw as charlatans who wanted to be like us but wouldn't take the risks, or for those who took too many risks simply for the thrill of it. There was deep friendship and even a bond of caring we could sometimes call love. We followed the wars and watered our sorrows, an endless season of adrenaline and alcohol.

The problems only came after we returned home, into a world that moved at a different pace, to people who lived the peaceful life I believe humans should live.

What was it like to live with such a man? I cannot and should not speak for the people who loved me. They are entitled to their own stories and memories of how it was, and to their privacy. But I can offer some accounting of myself. I was distant, far away in my thoughts, always planning the next escape to war when I should have been at ease among those who gave me every support and consideration. I did try hard to stay sober, and could succeed for months at a time. But I always went back. In the parlance of AA, I kept a seat reserved at the bar.

Success spurred denial. I rationalised: Yes, I was a drunk once upon a time, but I was in control now. How could I be winning awards from BAFTA, the Royal Television Society and all the rest, if I was really an alcoholic? The 1990s were the decade of prizes and herograms, of tempting job offers, and drinks with network bosses, a feast of praise and transient glories.

I lived two lives. The life of the road, where I could drink without anyone really noticing, and the life of home, where I struggled not to drink. How pathetic it seems to me now – gargling mouthwash and munching mints to kill the smell of booze, fooling nobody because nothing smells of alcoholism more than mints and mouthwash. I cannot think of those days without feeling more sorrow than I can ever express for the pain I caused with my addict's selfishness. That doesn't get forgotten, or written out.

10

The Fires Are Everywhere

'Why are you drinking?' asked the little prince.
'So that I may forget,' replied the drunkard.
'Forget what?' inquired the little prince, who already was sorry
    for him.
'Forget that I am ashamed,' the drunkard confessed, hanging
    his head.

Antoine de Saint-Exupéry[1]

It ran ahead of me, pulling me along a path full of slipping and falling with only dread at the end, morning after morning, wherever I was.

I will be good today.

I will not pick up.

Just use my will.

When the others break out the beers I will go to my room with a book.

But always defeat, the yielding of will and the same result. By the end of the 1990s the last vestiges of my control over alcohol were vanishing. It took a war to bring my drinking crisis to a head.

In early 1999 I was sent to the Balkans to cover the aftermath of the war in Bosnia and the looming crisis in Kosovo, where ethnic Albanians were being targeted by Serb police and paramilitaries at the behest of Slobodan Milošević. Bosnia now had an international peace agreement, foreign troops to protect it, and was, in effect, a ward of the international community. I had been in Africa for the years of the Balkan wars themselves, but Ireland and, in a much more marked way, the Rwandan genocide, gave me some sense of the emotions and manipulations which drove communal violence.

On my first night in Sarajevo, I got drunk in a bar run by an ex-policeman from Ireland. He had come to work with the international police force immediately after the war ended in 1995

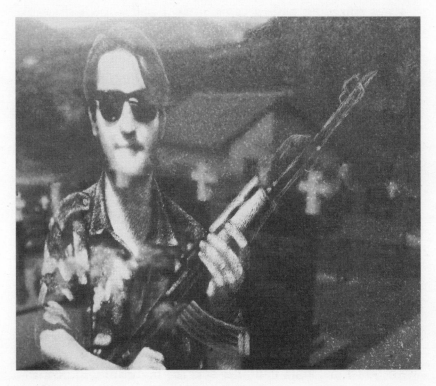

Serb grave, Bosnia.

and stayed on when his contract ended. He had slipped his moorings to the world back home. That night I got into an argument with another Irishman, an army officer on peacekeeping duties, about the rights and wrongs of the Balkan wars. He took the view that 'they are all as bad as each other' and, fuelled by drink, I became angry. I asked if he had ever been to war, rather than the aftermath. Had he seen death and maiming up close and what happened when politicians roused their people to hatred? He said that he had not. The conversation petered out. He was embarrassed. I had humiliated him. Even in drink, I knew there was no need for me to act as I had. I was losing my grip and lashing out where I could. The sanctimonious, drink-fuelled reporter is never a pleasant interlocutor.

I was travelling with a cameraman I had known since my Belfast days. Eugene McVeigh drank moderately but he didn't criticise me. 'We all have our off nights,' he said. We drank up and went back to the hotel. The following morning I woke to a grey winter city still gouged with the wounds of artillery and sniper fire from the war that had recently ended. Our assignment was to head north towards Tuzla on the trail of newly discovered mass graves.

We drove past empty villages, their occupants murdered, driven out, houses burned, roofless and graffitied. They were still digging out the big graves and the small: the ones filled with victims of massacres that the world would remember – Srebrenica, Višegrad, Zvornik – and those the world could not, small places in the mountains and valleys where neighbour had killed neighbour. I didn't know it then, but the trip had a dark resonance for Eugene. It would become apparent in the days ahead.

The grave at Donja Glumina held the bodies of 240 people – Muslim victims of ethnic cleansing from the start of the war in

1992. They had been buried by the Serb-controlled JNA (the Yugoslav National Army) who had used bulldozers to gouge deep trenches in a green field above the village. The bodies had recently been disinterred and taken to the mortuary in Tuzla, where families with missing relatives could inspect what remained of the dead. They were spraying the body bags, still caked with the mud of the grave, with disinfectant when we arrived. The jet of water sent the muddy ooze flying everywhere. The contents of each bag were then removed and laid out on top of the plastic: boots, scraps of clothes, a wallet, an insulin needle, spectacles, prayer beads, a skeletal hand. The smell was high and bitter, a mix of the lime the killers had used to speed up decomposition, and the residual rot of decaying bodies.

Eugene passed me some Vicks VapoRub and I stuffed my nose with the eucalyptus-scented ointment. He filmed quietly, keeping a respectful distance from the men with the hoses.

Inside the mortuary there was more cleaning. Jackets, shirts, jeans, scraps mostly, were being washed. The families might recognise what their loved one had been wearing on the day they disappeared. It is the kind of picture that can stay in the mind forever. There was a break in the afternoon and a boy brought beer and kebabs from the town. The cleaners gathered a short distance from the dead and ate their lunch. I assumed they were veterans of this kind of work. Then they resumed and kept going into the dark. There was still much to do, and the families of the dead would be arriving early in the morning.

Back at the hotel I showered and changed. But my skin felt impregnated by the reek of the dead. I could think only of getting a drink. Tomorrow would be worse yet I felt it was essential to be there. Although we had filmed the cleaning of the remains, mass murder without grief was absurd. All the time in this work, bidden or not, we intruded on the mourning of others. Would the relatives object to our presence? Most people either welcomed us at funerals or else were indifferent, too lost in their grief to pay attention to us. Only those with an instinctive mistrust of the media – loyalist paramilitaries in Belfast, for example – ever threatened us at funerals.

In the bar I praised Eugene for his sensitivity at the mortuary. We'd both found the experience traumatic. We spoke about back home and the people disappeared by the IRA into graves from which there was no returning to families and the sacred rituals for the dead. Then Eugene shared something personal. It was a story of family, Ireland and war, but most of all a story of trauma, the kind for which no medication or therapy can ever offer a definitive resolution. Back in 1975, his younger brother Columba (the name means 'Dove' in Gaelic) had moved to Dublin where Eugene was working as a cameraman for Irish television. It was a departure of necessity. The boy was seventeen and had been arrested by the RUC Special Branch after the army found bullets in a cigarette packet in the family home. The McVeighs strongly suspect it was a plant designed to pressurise Columba to infiltrate the IRA and become an informer. This was by no means a fanciful suspicion, given the dirtiness of the war between the IRA and the security forces during the 1970s.

Columba was remanded in jail and immediately came under suspicion from IRA prisoners. He was beaten up. When he was released – without charge – the suspicion intensified. He was harassed on the streets by the army and the IRA. In the end it got so bad that his parents advised him to go south. That was in the late summer of 1975. He disappeared on 1 November that same year. He just vanished. There was nothing to indicate who had taken him, no statement from any group. But nobody close to the story doubted that the IRA was responsible. There were plenty of rumours put out by 'Republican sources'. They claimed Columba had been killed after confessing during interrogation to being an informer. Interrogation in IRA terms usually meant torture: beatings, cigarette burns to the body. A gentle seventeen-year-old like Columba in the hands of hardened killers would likely have admitted to anything. The presumption was that Columba had been shot and then taken to a wood or a bog and buried. The IRA had been disappearing bodies into bogs since my grandparents' time.

I apologised to Eugene for bringing him to Tuzla. If I had known, I told him, I would never have inflicted this on him. There was no need for apology, he said. Work was work. It was his job and it mattered to him to record what had happened here. We spoke only of facts. I mostly listened. I did not need to ask him whether he experienced trauma over what happened to his little brother. There was no way the family could ever stop looking for him. They would never let the leaders of the Republican movement rest.

It was cold and misty the following morning. Relatives were gathering on the road outside the mortuary when we arrived just after eight. The shuffled through the gates. As they went in there were cries and gasps. The remains had been laid out in long lines with pathways between each. I saw, despite the decomposition, the open jaws of men who must have died screaming. The mothers, fathers, sisters and brothers of the missing paused before the different remains, sometimes pausing to inspect, moving on or staying because they might have recognised something: a piece of familiar clothing, an insulin needle, a pair of broken glasses. People were starting to recognise their dead. Some shouted. Some became hysterical. A girl cried 'Mustapha, Mustapha', then fell to the ground. Two women were helping an old man who was beside himself with sorrow. He collapsed onto a chair and a doctor came to examine him. His name was Rifat Osmanovic and he had found what was left of the body of his son.

After Tuzla, Eugene went back to his life in Ireland and to the family's campaign for truth. His mother, Vera, kept hoping Columba would come home alive, that maybe he had vanished overseas to live under an assumed name. In 1999, a year after our trip to Tuzla, the IRA finally admitted killing him, and she had to change focus. Now she wanted him home so that he could be buried among his own people. There were searches of bogland near the border between the Republic and Northern Ireland. The former IRA commander and Sinn Féin leader, Martin McGuinness, was even asked to help. But Columba was never found. Vera died in 2007 without knowing where her son lay.

As spring pulled towards summer the Balkans ignited again. This time Milošević dispatched his paramilitaries and police to deport the restive Albanians of Kosovo. I saw the war developing and longed to be there. I was not an old Balkan hand like many of my friends – journalists whose lives would be forever shaped by the experiences of Sarajevo and Srebrenica. Many of them were heading towards Kosovo in anticipation of witnessing the last act in Slobodan Milošević's murderous career.

Getting into Kosovo itself would have involved travelling secretly across the border with the Kosovo Liberation Army, and I had promised my family I would not risk death at the hands of Serb paramilitaries. I was capable of periods of lucidity. Instead I reported on the developing refugee crisis.

By the beginning of May 1999 around 600,000 people had fled Kosovo, crossing the borders of Albania and Macedonia to seek safety. As many as 400,000 more were displaced inside the country. I saw the long convoys of people crossing the border into Albania. They came on foot, dragging suitcases, or riding their tractors, or in coaches and beaten-up old cars. There was one car in which the driver, a man in his middle age, sat crying. He covered his face with a blanket to hide the tears from his family and from me. I stepped back from the car. His wife motioned me to return. 'The fires are everywhere,' she said.

There were two children sitting in the back. The younger one leaned forward and put his hand on his dad's shoulder. He left it there for a few minutes, and when the traffic began to inch forward, squeezed gently before sitting back once more.

Another day I was on the border watching the smoke rise from NATO airstrikes on Serb positions, and a van pulled up with a wounded man and his wife and several children. He had been shot in the leg. The man was transferred to an ambulance. When the boy saw his father being taken away, he screamed and screamed, and became hysterical. His mother and some other relatives moved in to hold him. The paramedics agreed that he could travel in the ambulance with his father.

The refugees slept in their vehicles, on the roadside, and in camps that were beginning to spring up outside the border town of Kukës. Those newly arrived were given blankets at a stall set up by the UN. Driving back down to the town I saw refugees being stopped by local thugs, and the blankets they had been given a few moments earlier were stolen. The people were too exhausted and frightened to complain. I wanted to get out and protest. A policeman got there before me, then backed away suddenly as the gang leader revealed a pistol.

Sixteen thousand refugees crossed into Kukës by the end of that weekend. Everywhere we went there were traumatised people. They told stories of killing and sexual violence. Trafficking gangs had already arrived in the town to abduct girls and young women.

I was part of the familiar flotsam of war. There were reporters still haunted by Croatia and Bosnia, hoping the moment had come when Milošević would finally be stopped. There were the aid workers from charities large and small, part of an industry that was multiplying exponentially in the last years of the century, diplomats and spooks, and some pretending to be one or the other, a medical team from the Israeli Defense Force, eager to boost the country's image, a contingent of army doctors from the United Arab Emirates who set up a camp that became legendary for its luxurious tents and good food.

Our BBC team rented a house, which became home to a family of refugees who arrived at the door asking for a place to sleep. The father went by the name of 'Easy' and was well named, a good-humoured chef from Mitrovica. With his wife, Easy established a domestic routine. They shopped and cooked and kept the house clean. In return we gave them food and shelter and access to our satellite phone to communicate with family still inside Kosovo. The two children, a girl aged seven and a boy aged four, filled the place with noise, sometimes laughter, other times squabbling. We adopted a dog, a scrawny three-legged creature we named Tripod.

We were an odd little community. But in Easy and his little tribe I detected a solidity. Despite what they had lost, the family was holding together. I never once saw him, or his wife, become bad-tempered or impatient, either with each other or with the children. I felt a reproach in this domestic solidity. It was what I craved, yet what I constantly ran from. There was nothing Easy wanted more than to be back at home in Mitrovica on the banks of the Ibar river, cooking meals for whoever came to his restaurant, back to the world that existed before hatred tore his city apart.

I was becoming unmoored from any emotional stability. In the last few months before Kosovo, I had been to Bosnia, Congo and Sierra Leone, and I was already thinking of where I might go next after the Balkan trip. Looking now at that list of destinations of the spring of 1999, all within weeks of each other, I return to that word which gives this book its name: madness. Not only the madness of what I saw, though it was abundant, but the deepening downward spiral within. It was there in the risks that I took and the alcohol I drank.

I put down now what I thought I had forgotten of those last days of my drinking life, rearing back at me in splashes of blood and tropical green and brown hillsides. As I ransack my memory the images trigger my senses: the smells of rotting jungle vegetation, of palm oil, of cheap cigarettes in a Macedonian bar, and voices that I have not heard in decades.

Freetown, March 1999

I see soldiers torture a man in the garden of my hotel. He is a fisherman. But they say he's been spying on military positions. They kick and punch him. I see a trickle of blood run down his neck. A rifle is cocked, and he screams in a way that I never imagined a human could scream, as if the voice has left his body, fled to a place of animal terror, echoing across the swimming pool to the Atlantic beyond. I do not intervene. The soldiers are volatile. People are constantly being accused of supporting the rebels. Summary executions are happening all over the city.

The man is hustled away, to his death I am convinced. But he reappears later. Perhaps the fact that I was watching as they took him away saved his life: there might be questions to their superiors from a meddling white man, a journalist. Or perhaps the soldiers believed his story, or he found a way to bribe them.

A few days later. I am walking with others in the BBC team down at the creek near the Aberdeen Bridge when we spot a body lying on the foreshore. We are escorted by two Nigerian peacekeepers. One is a brute whom I have seen beat a woman at a checkpoint. The other seems more sensitive and speaks of his dreams of studying sociology at college. The body is a man's, a mess of bruises and welts. His hands have been tied behind his back. Whoever killed him has not spared the torture. There are five gunshot wounds in his back. The more articulate soldier says, 'That will teach him for being a rebel.' The oaf kicks the body. Tiny crabs scuttle away.

Some children pass by on the road above us, three of them – an older girl of about ten, and two young boys. They glance down but do not stop. By the standards of Freetown today there is nothing very unusual in what they witness. Besides, they know how the 'peacekeepers' can be. In the wrong mood they might beat a child who stops to stare.

I go to Paddy's Bar, overlooking the lagoon, to drink among the prostitutes and the mercenaries and aid workers and journalists, all of us feeding off the war and – in ways I do not yet understand – being consumed in return. The mercenaries fly the gunships that keep the rebels at bay. There's Neil Ellis, a veteran of South Africa's border wars, and Fijian Fred, who's ex-SAS and, as his nickname suggests, comes from Fiji.

Neil doesn't shy away from journalists like some mercenaries do. He is one of those restless men caught on the wrong side of history when the white regimes of Rhodesia, where he grew up and fought, and then South Africa, were replaced by Black majority rule. Many go from war to war in Africa. Soon the wars in Afghanistan and Iraq will offer new opportunities for men who no longer have the countries of their youth. War is their nation now. 'I have not been paid for twenty months,' Neil tells an interviewer. 'I do it because I don't know what else to do. I enjoy the excitement. It's an adrenaline rush.'[2] Fred's real name is Kauta Marafono, and by the time I meet him he has been fighting for more than three decades, a bear of a man who wields the door gun on Neil Ellis's helicopter, and who has gone through two marriages because he can never settle at home.

After returning from blasting rebels into eternity, Neil and Fred fly low over the bar to announce their imminent arrival. It is the daily signal to get the beers ready. Neil and Fred keep the rebels from overrunning Freetown and murdering the population. In a place full of homicidal men and boys, the rebels of the RUF – Revolutionary United Front – terrify us more than anyone. The RUF leaders have names like 'Rambo Red Goat', 'Captain Blood' and 'Bomb Blast', and they are chopping off hundreds of limbs – mostly arms and hands, because these are what people use to vote. In the bar one night a man called Roy, a local militia fighter, tells me how he saw a three-year-old boy hung upside down from a tree while a rebel tried to hack off his head with a machete. The rebel succeeded before Roy could shoot him.

Years later I read a court report that says the killing and torture was designed to 'instil terror in the civilian population'.[3] Maybe that was the case at the start but for me, then, it seemed to have its own remorseless logic, a horror movie fantasy from the brutalised minds of child soldiers flooding directly into the minds of their traumatised victims, a cottage industry of death and mayhem keeping the UN, countless NGOs, mercenaries and yours truly and his comrades employed in our own circus of rescuers, fighters, witnesses and also, occasionally, victims. There is a murderous energy vibrating through jungle and city, the ghosts of colonialism and slavery ricocheting endlessly out of the past, the never-ending bequest of poverty and misrule, and, always, white men gorging on the oil, the blood diamonds, the platinum, the coltan, the uranium; white men in helicopters with guns, white men with their bought-off African politicians; those other white men and women with their unending need to be good and to be seen to be good, hawking their compassion from one African Calvary to the next, with their aid programmes and four-by-fours, fleets of them as far as the eye can see; and you will find me there too, gifted with the privilege of cynicism, a lame laureate of misery burning fast and out towards some end I cannot see. Yes, I am at home here. The beers are flowing and the sounds of the war drift across the lagoon.

The owner of Paddy's Bar is an elderly Irishman who came out to Sierra Leone in colonial times and managed to keep a bar running through coup and counter coup. He is kindly and gives a home to a crew of refugees and orphans, who cook and clean and serve beer to those who crowd under his palm roof. He briefly fell foul of the prostitutes when he tried to ban them after a big fight between the local women and the Liberians, who tried to move in on their territory. The drama erupted on the night of a birthday dinner for the Italian ambassador. Peace was restored with promises of good behaviour.

This phase of the war has already killed several of our clan. My Sierra Leonian BBC colleague Edward Smith was shot dead the previous year, and ten other local journalists brutally murdered when the rebels attacked Freetown at the start of January 1999.

The American journalist, Myles Tierney, was killed in the middle of that mayhem. He was travelling in a convoy with the Minister of Information when they were ambushed. The conflict would take two more the following year: Kurt Schork, one of the great reporters of the siege of Sarajevo, and Gil Moreno, a long, lean Spaniard I encountered in the Balkans. Death could come for you in Sierra Leone no matter how experienced you were. My old friend from the South African township days, Mark Chisholm, and a Greek colleague, Yannis Behrakis, were caught in the ambush that killed Schork and Moreno but escaped and fled into the bush, wandering separately in terror for their lives, until they were rescued by an army patrol. Chisholm remembers that in the last seconds before the ambush he knew something was not right. The road was too quiet. He wanted to turn back.

We drink until dusk begins to creep up, and then head back to the hotel. Not even the mercenaries want to risk facing a check-point after dark when a scared teenager with an AK-47 might mistake you for an enemy, or a ghost.

Kukës, May 1999

My nights in Kukës develop a numbing routine. I drink on my own. Avoiding colleagues, I then head out onto the streets, past the families sleeping in the open, and wonder what is happening in the other, sane world in which my wife and child are living, guilty for being away from them but unable to stop.

Back at the house I keep drinking until I fall asleep.

My rotation ends with the arrival of warmer weather. Summer is coming. The NATO bombing campaign against the Serbs is beginning to reverse the course of the war. Soon it might be possible for Easy and all the others to go back to Kosovo.

My last memory of the war is a ride in a helicopter taking me on the first leg of the journey to London. We cross snow-capped mountains. I look down and, in brilliant sunshine, see a bear scampering across a ridge. For a few seconds I feel something like pleasure. The beauty of that mountain scene pushes me out of myself. I am flying home to go away again – to begin a holiday with some friends – a journey that will end with a confrontation I had never anticipated.

11

Terms of Surrender

By the ways of Cangas
The voice of the wind moaned:
Alas, how lonely you have remained.

'María Soliña', traditional Galician ballad[1]

I am a week or so out of Kosovo, and we are driving along the northern coast of Spain, a landscape that reminds me of the west coast of Ireland with its cliffs and rocky promontories. The others have gone to dinner. They are three good friends from Ireland – a marine biologist, a priest, and a policeman. Each has known me for many years. They are people with big hearts. If ever there is a group of individuals with whom I should feel able to share my feelings it is these. None has any connection to journalism or war.

We drive into the mountains of Galicia, on the way south to Santiago de Compostela, along the Way of St James, a route of Christian pilgrimage since the eleventh century. But we eschew the hardships of blistered feet and weary limbs suffered by the walkers we pass along the high mountain roads. There are days of cold rainy mornings and afternoon sunlight. We stop in small villages to wander and eat and drink.

Occasionally I catch sight of a news bulletin on a pub television. The NATO raids in Kosovo are escalating. The Serbs are retreating. My instinct is to call the holiday short and go back. I telephone my boss in London and offer to get on the next plane. 'Take it easy,' he says, 'there'll be plenty war left for you to go back to in a week.'

I cannot bear the idea of missing the finale, yet I am in too poor a state from drinking to do any kind of work. I wake up hungover every day, my head battered from the inside, my stomach feeling as if it has been scoured by a steel pad. On the ship coming over, I developed an agonising abscess in my tooth. The doctor on board gave me codeine and warned me not to drink alcohol. I drank and was sick as the boat pitched and bumped through the Bay of Biscay.

At Santiago de Compostela I establish a routine of waking after a few hours of broken sleep, heading out of the hotel room I share with my friend the priest, and wandering to a little park I have found where I can drink from my bottle of whiskey. The bottle comes with me everywhere, hidden at the bottom of a shoulder bag – my medicine. I am terrified now. There is no stopping this compulsion. Do the others notice? If they do, they have decided individually or collectively to say nothing.

I always come back in time for breakfast, my breath smothered with peppermint, trying to give the impression of a man on holiday. I count the hours to lunchtime when I can drink and my drinking will look normal, part of the routine of people travelling and having fun together. The space between my dawn whiskey and the first beer at midday becomes a hell. No amount of mint chewing-gum can rid my mouth of the taste of bile. By the end of the week, I am isolating from my friends, just as I had isolated myself in Kukës. Only in this way can I drink in the way that I need to.

I have been through blackouts, the compulsion, the shame, the lying, the hangovers, the depression, but have always found a way to stop for a while, or at least ease off. Now there is no stopping. Never has alcohol made me feel so afraid. The substance which I have used to medicate the symptoms of trauma has become the problem.

I am back in London. It is early morning. My little attic study is hot and airless. I have been up all night. I indulge the self-pity that is common to so many alcoholics – *poor me, poor me, pour me another*. But I cannot, will not take a drink. Something stops me from going to the cabinet and taking out a bottle. I veer from need to need. I want to be rescued. I do not want to be rescued. I want to be left alone. I wish somebody would knock at the door. My family is away in Ireland. I am physically, mentally and morally exhausted. The old cure no longer works. A phone call from a close family member, speaking simple words of concern, calling me to reality, brings me the final yards to an acceptance of defeat. It is over. I promise those I love that I will stop drinking, and that having been said I feel in the pit of my stomach that I am at last telling the truth. I believe myself. There can be no going back.

I never believed I belonged in rehab, a 'headcase drunk' washed up in one of those places where I'd seen my father – marooned among the shamefaced and scared while his son mingled with the visitors: the angry, frightened husbands and wives, the embarrassed children, and me wanting to run out the gates to the world of normal people. There always seemed to be an intrusive counsellor urging me to get more involved in my father's recovery, as if all that was needed was for me to sit and recite his failings in one of those brutal family groups where everybody ended up crying or shouting, all in the name of breaking the drunkard's denial. It was shock therapy, the alcoholic's boot camp. I always left feeling as though my father had been somehow reduced. It didn't save him. How would it save me?

But in that summer in 1999 I am ready to do anything to stop drinking.

I call a friend whose seventy-eight-year-old mother had treatment and has been three years sober. He recommends a specific hospital: 'If she can do it, then you can.'

I then call my boss and tell him I must get help. He doesn't say too much except that I should work on being well, and to take as much time as I need. 'The work you do takes its toll,' he adds. 'Your job will be waiting for you.'

I pack a bag and call a taxi. In that moment nothing of what has gone before, not all my father's journeys through the detox and rehab units of Ireland, my resentment of the counsellors and doctors, make any difference. I just feel an overwhelming sense of relief.

At the hospital I sign forms and submit to a blood test to see if there is any booze in my system. If there is a high blood-alcohol level you get sedatives to help the come-down. Alcoholics in the advanced stages of a spree can get fatal seizures if they aren't properly weaned off the booze.

I have done my own cold turkey full of sweats and shaking at home and don't need medication. They search my clothes and bags. Some people find it humiliating. I do not. My pride has puked itself up too many times along the way for me to bridle at this intrusion. For the first time in many years, I feel physically safe. From war, from myself.

The world outside does not matter at that moment. My personal space has contracted dramatically. There is my small room overlooking the garden. There is the chapel where the AA meetings are held. There is the room on the other side of the compound where we go for group therapy each day, and another smaller room for one-to-one sessions with counsellors. There is the canteen where, three times a day, the alcoholics sit together to complain, cry, laugh, and hold each other. There are people here because they've been forced in – by the legal system, through family intervention, by an ultimatum from work. Some in that category want to be outside and using, so they hide a bottle or a stash of drugs in their bags, or arrange for visitors to bring some in and hide it in their room or the grounds. There are regular searches for contraband. The deal is that if you get caught drinking or using you are out. No appeals.

On my first evening, I sit in a room full of alcoholics and drug addicts. Three things abound: remorse, shame and denial. The men and women in the group are a mix of British and foreigners, of different social classes, and addictions that range from alcohol and drugs (the majority) to gambling, spending and sex, and a few with mixes of all five – the platinum class of the addicts' world. A group leader is chosen by acclamation. Later, when we are halfway through the twenty-eight-day programme, there is another election. I think I might be chosen. I'd spent the previous week joking with and charming people. But I guess my neediness is too obvious. Or they spot someone who might want too much to lead and control. I am not even considered. That is the first lesson in humility. Many more will follow.

When we complain to staff about the food or the structure of the day, or occasionally about a particular staff member, we are reminded that we are in hospital out of choice. 'This is not a summer camp,' the lead counsellor declares. 'This is a psychiatric hospital. That is where you are. You are in a PSYCHIATRIC HOSPITAL.'

The counsellors operate from the basis that most people who come in the door are more, or less, in denial. We are told that we are lucky to be there. Most alcoholics never get to rehab. We are told that 30 per cent relapse in their first year of sobriety, but if we stick it out for a year the chances of relapse drop by half.

At least five of the thirty or so of those who were in the room with me in the early days are dead now, from drinking or drug overdoses.

The system in rehab works to create a group bond, so that we learn to reach out, to trust others (always a big struggle with addicts) and to be dependable (an even greater struggle). There are film stars and street addicts, and business people who've succumbed to the late twentieth-century epidemic of cocaine addiction.

What are you in for?

Charlie

And you?

The booze.

From these basic beginnings many fruitful conversations follow. There are slogans on the walls of the rooms where we gather for our group meetings. In another time, in my years of denial, I would have cynically dismissed them. Now, I write out the slogans on paper and stick them up in my room. They are the first thing I see when I wake.

Easy Does It.

FEAR – Face Everything and Recover.

This Too Shall Pass.

One Day at a Time.

A lot of our group struggle with the idea of handing their troubles over to a so-called 'Higher Power'. I decide early on I won't let my mistrust of religion get in the way of sobriety. I will leave religion, as it operated in the Ireland of my childhood, out of the equation. As for the Higher Power ... I am so screwed up and afraid I'd give the family cat that role and hope for the best.

'A Higher Power can be anything you want,' one of the counsellors says. 'The idea is to get rid of the impulse to control everything. You cannot control your drinking. You wouldn't be here if you could ... Hand it over and trust things will be okay.'

I think of a story a friend in Ireland told me. He had taken me to my very first AA meeting in the 1980s and was trying to explain the Higher Power concept. Joe was a Corkman and, like myself, a survivor of the repressive Catholicism of childhood, with an inbuilt aversion to organised religion. When he rocked up in rehab the counsellors struggled to get him to engage. 'It's not religion, Joe,' one told him. 'It's just a way of getting you to take the pressure off yourself. Hand over the fear and resentment to someone else.'

'Higher Power? That is fucking religion.'

'No, it is not.'

Then, a flash of Corkish wit brought Joe over the line. 'No offence to you personally,' he told his interlocutor, 'but if I believed in that shite I would be going against all I stand for. I would be a hypocrite. A bloody hypocrite.'

To which he received the following response: 'Joe, I don't mean to insult you, but I need to give it to you straight. You are here because you cannot stop drinking, you are constantly messing up your life, you steal from those who love you ... At this moment you are a fuckin' degenerate. Hypocrite would be a step up in the world for you.'

Joe was many years sober when we met.

* * *

In rehab I read widely about addiction, not only tracts about the '12 Steps' – the route map to sobriety for those who quit drinking – but books about the science of addiction, and the links between addiction and different kinds of mental illness. I read how alcohol hooked me into an endless cycle of chemical dependency, constantly setting up my body to fail and fall again. It is hard to convey to the non-addicted the relief in learning that alcoholism is not caused by moral weakness, however much it distorts the moral personality of the addict.

We repeat the slogan: *We are not bad people trying to become good. We are sick people trying to become well.* This isn't some kind of confessional, get-off-scot-free clause for past bad behaviour. In each life there are reckonings and atonements. But starting to purge the poison of self-hatred is an essential beginning.

A week into my treatment I meet Gordon Duncan. I loathe him pretty instantly. Until he becomes one of my best friends, and certainly the man who comes to know me better than any other.

Like most of our counsellors Gordon is a former alcoholic/ addict. He's come to counselling by way of several different lives. He's owned a fishing trawler, been a bookie, and a publican. Gordon is tall, stocky, balding, blunt-spoken and disinclined to social niceties – a man whose social outlook in many ways belongs to the vanished world of the big talkers and bigger spenders he met in the pubs and on the racetracks of the flash 1960s. He mistrusts credit cards and always carries large wads of cash to pay his way.

Gordon does not speak in the late twentieth-century language of therapy – there is no urging that I commune with my 'inner child' – but what he says he always means, and when it comes to alcoholism he is unfailingly right. It is Gordon who identifies my anger in a group therapy session and gives me the first tools to deal with it: *Step back, count to ten, breathe deeply; ask yourself what is really happening inside you; walk away if the anger is going to overwhelm. Say sorry. Say it as often as you need to. You are stronger than you think.* When he dies in 2015, I mourn a man who had become a substitute father to me. In his last days, I sat by his bed in Kingston Hospital, hoping that he could hear me as he drifted away. I whispered into his ear, again and again, the words of the Serenity Prayer. From Gordon I had begun to learn the difference between what I could change, and what I could not.

Until rehab I had never thought of myself as angry. My social interactions – drunk or sober – were usually peaceful. I'd constructed a whole persona out of being the warm, charming Irish guy. It wasn't a lie. It just wasn't the whole truth. I did not get into physical fights in bars, but if I felt under verbal attack I wanted to crush opposition before it might crush me. I also withdrew into silences, building a wall that flashed a warning: *Cross me, complain to me, ask anything of me and I will retreat even further. See how you like that. Leave me alone. Alone.*

I have a memory of shouting at a producer in Singapore, while we were on the trail of a crook who always seemed to be one step ahead of the pursuing media. I was tired, hungover, under pressure – oh excuses, excuses – and what should have been a polite request to focus on the job rather than go around in circles was expressed as a belligerent roar. I remember the faces of the others in our small group, people I worked with all the time, their expressions asking: *Where in the fuck did that come from?*

In the unpredictable spaces of group therapy, sitting among other angry addicts, where anything might be said by anyone, there was no way of hiding my anger.

I had begun therapy by trying to be the best recovering alcoholic in the hospital. I'd read all the literature promptly. I filled in the questionnaires before anybody else. At night I listened to the sad stories of others and offered sage advice. As one of my contemporaries later wrote to me: 'I got to like you, but only after you stopped pretending you were actually one of the counsellors who had been put among the addicts as some kind of secret operation.' I badly wanted sobriety, but I was less enthusiastic about opening myself up to the judgements of my fellow patients.

Every one of us in that place had a persona we presented to the world. And most of us were angry with old wounds and abandonments.

Gordon used to say that my brain would be the death of me. 'You spend your life thinking, living in your fucking head. Get out into the real world, Fergal.'

Midway through the twenty-eight-day programme we are expected to write the story of our lives. This is to be an accounting, in unflinching detail, of our paths to alcoholism. Nothing is to be left out.

I have spent my life telling the stories of others, with all the tricks at a writer's disposal. This testament has to be written out by hand, however. We are not allowed computers. I think the idea is to have one less tool of potential evasion between us and the truth.

If I want to get better, Gordon tells me, I will have to describe every low move, every lie, every shameful incident, all that cannot be told anywhere else, or in front of anybody else. 'Shame is a killer,' he says, 'but no matter how shameful you think your past is there is always someone, maybe even one of your counsellors, who can top it.'

If this public accounting had been described to me before coming in, I'd have dismissed the whole exercise as Maoist self-criticism with a twist of psychobabble. But I couldn't maintain that cynical shield with Gordon on my case. He told me I couldn't do what he referred to as 'my writer bullshit' ... No fine words ... 'A to fucking B and all the way to Z. Write it all out.' And not simply a catalogue of infamies. 'Talk about how you tried to stop drinking. Talk about the decent and good in you as well. That guy never went away.'

The week before my own story I sit through the reading of an artist with whom I've made friends. Here is a man I know as a gifted individual, but he reads now in a low murmur I do not recognise. When he has finished, he folds into sobs, his body rocking back and forth. Afterwards there is silence and then some sharing: respectful, caring, conscious of the immense effort it has taken him to come to this point. By now we all want each other to be well. Never before, and never since, have I experienced the power of a small community working all of their waking hours to help one another in something that was ultimately, if followed to the most logical of conclusions, a matter of life and death.

When my turn comes, I feel at first as if the silence in the room will overwhelm me. Here is an audience I cannot seduce. My hands are shaking. But I look into the faces of those with whom I have already worked so hard, and I understand that I don't need to catch and reel them in. The faces looking back at me want me well. We are a fellowship.

I say what has happened. There are people here who know me from my public life, who even told me how much they liked my work when I came in to rehab. Well, now they are getting an alternative version. I don't remember ever feeling so exposed.

When it is done, I do not cry but feel an immense exhaustion. I sit back in my chair and let the relief flow over me.

Afterwards my friends come up and hug me. My people. The drunks, junkies and chancers, the fly-by-nights, the dreamers, the refugees from themselves – all of us safe in that place for some precious weeks in the last summer of the century.

I think I knew then that if I worked at this I could stay sober. There was no magic code to crack. At its most fundamental my philosophy each day was *Just don't pick up a drink. When the craving comes pick up a phone, talk to another alcoholic, go to a meeting with other recovering drunks. Go to a meeting.*

They were some of the happiest days in my life. The world had stopped. I could feel myself getting stronger. I had, as the phrase goes, been unchained from my personal alcoholic lunatic. There were people in there with me who were on their second and third rehabs. The counsellors would tell them that they couldn't afford to give up hope. Somehow they found the strength to try again. *Always get up and clean yourself up and try once more, and ask yourself: do I want to die from this thing?*

For some the pain was too deep to shift. It was part of the skin and soul of who they were. A thousand rehabs wouldn't save them. They went through the motions, for bosses, or lovers and family. And then, after a few days, even a few hours, they would head to the pub, the off-licence, or straight into the grateful embrace of their dealer. I cannot judge them. They were people who, through telling their stories, helped me put one foot in front of the other and keep walking.

The founders of AA described those who fail to achieve sobriety as people who are constitutionally incapable of being honest with themselves. I have always thought there is more to terminal addiction than that. I am careful to remember that for all the universality of symptoms, each addict's pain is a personal mystery. The solutions might be available to all, but I am no nearer understanding now than I was when I first became sober, what allowed me to 'get' sobriety and why my father could not. It was not because he lacked the desire, or that he had not suffered enough, or could not count the cost of it all.

There is an incident towards the end of my twenty-eight days which shocks everyone and blows away the 'pink cloud' – the sense of infinite possibility that is the frequent experience of those in their early days of sobriety.

A young man I will call James had been with us from the start. He was a junkie who first became addicted to heroin in the 1980s when the drug swept through the council estates of his native city in the north of England. Over the weeks I'd watched him confront his past. At weekends I saw him play with his seven-year-old daughter on the lawn in front of the hospital. The girl was sullen and withdrawn at first. She resisted her father's embraces. There had been too many vanishings for her to trust. She had been to see him in other hospitals.

Each time the same thing happened. He made it a few days and then relapsed. When James stuck a needle in his arm he sank in plain sight. The child had seen him passed out on the floor being revived by paramedics. She knew what dealers looked like: they were furtive, never-hang-around-too-long, never meet-your-gaze type of young men selling gear for the bigger fish; they were junkie-dealers who limped because they stuck needles in the veins in their legs, and because they were not paid enough to fund their own habits sometimes ripped off the suppliers and ended up getting battered or dying. They were something that couldn't be washed out of the family's life as long as her dad was using. The idea was that the hospital in London would get him away from the heroin swamp back home.

James would come to our nightly group meeting and wonder if winning back his daughter's trust wasn't just a waste of time. *No, no, we would reassure him, it would come right in the end.* After the meeting ended, we'd go outside and drink tea and coffee and play music, and James would be gathered in by this group of one-time no-hopers who had found in each other a place of safety.

The third weekend in there was a change in his daughter. She smiled. She leaned her head against him when they picnicked on the grass. The dad she came to see was a different dad. James was alert and attentive and able to be in one place without always looking off into the distance.

He was happy that night, happier than I had seen him since we first met. The following morning I was walking with my artist friend and we came across James standing in the driveway with his bags. He said he was going home. When he talked he looked at the ground; his voice was not the open voice of the man in the group sessions or talking football on the lawn under the stars, singing along to the Rolling Stones's 'Tumbling Dice'.

The artist asked him to stay. 'You've only got another week to go to finish this thing.'

'Don't give up so close,' I said.

He told us he would go to Narcotics Anonymous meetings. He was strong enough now to resist. There was some stuff he wanted to sort and anyway it was time to get back into caring for his daughter.

'I know you are going to see a dealer,' I said.

No, no, he said. Back and forth we went. And then he said, yes. It was just too fucking hard. His child would be better without him in her life.

You can beg an addict not to use but it won't work, because when they have that fucked-up guttering candle look in their eyes, no force on earth short of tying them up and sticking them in a padded cell will stop them using. We embraced him. I don't know what the taxi driver thought when he pulled into the hospital driveway and saw three grown men huddled together and then one of them trying to pull away and the others not letting go. Until the artist and I knew there was no point. James threw his bag onto the back seat of the taxi, stepped in and drove away, not looking back to wave or say goodbye, but feeling the immense pull that was carrying him to his future outside our cocooned and sober world.

I heard from another junkie who had managed to reach James one night that he was back on the smack and living in a squat. That was the end of it. I never heard of him again.

Every one of us knew the territory. People could look as if they really had it beaten and a day later be hammered out of their mind and a week after that in intensive care or found dead in their flat. Another of our core mantras was that addiction was *cunning, baffling and powerful*. It was patient. It would wait until your defences were down and then strike. I knew from the past when I had periods of sobriety that I never suddenly decided to pick up a drink. The plan was always formed weeks before. It would start with a mental picture of a beer or a whiskey or a glass of wine. The image would quickly translate into a feeling of anticipation, so that I began to taste the beer-sweet and whiskey-sting on my lips, the relief of booze hitting the bloodstream. The cravings would accelerate until I cracked.

* * *

Gordon talked about the idea of the 'yets'.

I hadn't lost my family to alcohol ... *yet*.

I hadn't lost my home ... *yet*.

I hadn't lost my job ... *yet*.

I hadn't lost my health ... *yet*.

'But if you want that,' said Gordon, 'it's waiting for you in technicolour glory, son. It's a guarantee. You will lose the fucking lot.'

In the 'rooms' where I go to meet other alcoholics after my release from hospital, there are people who inspire me, and people I can't stand. There are men and women of hard-earned wisdom and humility, and know-alls and false messiahs looking for a stage. I work at keeping my judgements to myself, and the harder I work the more I succeed. I figure if I am damned with this compulsive nature I might as well use it to save my life.

Gordon becomes my permanent one-to-one counsellor. Every week we spend an hour talking through what is bothering me. Giving up the chemical connection between pain and temporary relief is the easy part. Dealing with the rioting emotions of this addict is the harder path. Sometimes I feel extraordinary physical exhaustion from the effort. One day, sitting opposite Gordon during a one-to-one therapy session, he says to me: 'You are too tired to make sense of anything, mate. Go into the garden and sit under the tree and sleep. It'll be a good use of our time.'

For all the struggle they involve, these early days of sobriety have the quality of a reverie in my memory. I am on sick leave from work. There is no pressure except the pressure to be well, and I can handle this. I embrace it.

Like so many alcoholics I drank on my resentments, topped up every time I became convinced that I was being abandoned, slighted or mistreated. I constantly felt betrayal was around the corner. It was exhausting to live this way. Exhausting for the alcoholic, even more so for those trying to love them. And if the active alcoholic can seem a self-obsessed individual, the recovering alcoholic, especially in early recovery, runs them a hard second. I wavered between excessive apologetics and angry withdrawal.

Still, I leave rehab with reasonable confidence that I can stay sober. I have plenty of support. My fellow recovering alcoholics are on standby if I begin to waiver. There are my meetings – ninety in ninety days, as the old-timers suggest – which make sobriety a daily way of life. Some friends fall by the wayside. Some come back to sobriety. Others get lost and never return. But I keep going. In this endeavour, at least, I am consistent.

About a year into this changed life I am offered a lesson. It comes in the form of another man's suffering. I am sure this is the point where I start thinking seriously about where trauma and addiction intersect. It happens because Gordon is encouraging me to help others who are struggling. 'To keep it, you've got to give it away,' he repeats. So he puts me on a list of people who have gone through rehab and are willing to help others trying to get sober.

One morning the hospital calls and asks if I will come and visit an old BBC colleague who is trying to beat an addiction to booze and cocaine. I haven't seen Bill Frost in the decade or so since he left the BBC. I use his real name here because his sister, Clare Campbell, wrote a memoir of his lonely death, hoping it might encourage other addicts to seek help.

Bill is a charming, raffish character who has reported from the wars in Lebanon and Bosnia, a fine writer and broadcaster who I looked up to in my early days at the BBC. But even in an atmosphere of notable tolerance for hard drinking, he stood out.

He still functioned, however, well enough for *The Times* newspaper to lure him away from the BBC to become its chief reporter.

I go to see him and come away shocked by his physical condition. The handsome, charismatic figure of a few years before is haggard and haunted. We talk about the stress of our work in war zones and about the boozing and drug-taking that has taken away several of our colleagues. He speaks of Bosnia and how his drinking and drug use escalated after the war. Bill really wants to be clean. I don't believe he says this to please me. I know how you can hold two competing, desperate desires at the same time. *I want to stop all this.* And *I want a fix.* Around and around. Until you surrender to one choice or the other, or the body gets there ahead of you and a ruined liver, a rotting pancreas, a broken heart – in the true, the literal sense – or any of the other grim possibilities of deep addiction make the choice for you.

Though I am still early in sobriety myself, I share with Bill a little of what has worked for me so far. We meet again a few times and speak by phone. Then the phone calls stop. Until one morning I wake up to a message that has been sent in the middle of the night. Bill wants to talk. He is struggling. I call back but it goes through to his voicemail. *If he's serious about getting clean he'll ring again*, I reason.

Not long after that, a few weeks maybe, I hear that Bill has been found dead in his flat. When an addict dies, I think of the sober life that might have been. I think of the pain that has laid them low. I think *There but for the Grace of God – or the clutch of luck, or the mysteries of the mind that allowed me to escape – go I.* There is a memorial service at St Bride's, the journalists' church on Fleet Street. We sing one of his favourite songs, the old ballad 'The Parting Glass'.

And all the harm that e're I've done
Alas it was to none but me.
And all I've done for want of wit
To mem'ry now I can't recall
So fill to me the parting glass
Goodnight and joy be with you all.[2]

The last months of his life were a descent into the worst kind of
drugged-up hell. Bill had begun a relationship with the sister of a
drug dealer. At various stages he had been given drugs, cash, and
weapons to hide in his home. In his chronically addicted and
increasingly paranoid state he was an easy mark for a big-time
dealer. Finally, his body gave out. At the age of forty-eight Bill
Frost died from an embolism – a blood clot in the lungs – caused
by cocaine abuse.

His sister Clare reflected on her brother's self-destructive path:
'Who really was to blame for his death? Drugs had done it for him,
but so had Bill's addictive personality that for so long had led him
to seek out risk and danger from Beirut to Bosnia. Perhaps [the
drug dealer's] doings provided a debased substitute for all of that.
It was as if, I began to think, Bill had found a substitute for war.'[3]

After getting sober I avoid war for nearly six months. Gordon says
I need a stable environment. There are to be no trips to places that
might trigger a desire for alcoholic escape. I work on a documentary series about marginalised communities in Britain. I go to
meet shipyard workers in Scotland, farmers in Wales and Cornwall
and families living on a drug-infested housing estate in Leeds.
These people are sometimes desperate and all are struggling, but
it is not war. After the day's filming I leave the others and meet
other recovering alcoholics wherever I am. It is a peaceful period

and, had I been able to grasp it then, a time when I might have changed course in journalism completely.

Long after I leave rehab I see my doctor's file from those early days of alcohol recovery. I am described as motivated and determined: 'His prospects for recovery are strong.' But there is something else in the notes. 'The patient is showing underlying symptoms of PTSD concurrent with his war experiences.'

If any doctor said anything about this to me at the time I don't remember. The purpose of my rehab was to stop alcohol addiction. Never in those twenty-eight days did I suggest to my counsellors that there was another addiction rebelling in my psyche. I was so far from such a realisation myself. I wanted to be sober, but I had no desire to give up my work in the zones of death.

It would take another twenty years, and much risk and anguish, before I came to the point of accepting that I was addicted to war.

12

Siege

Watch out or fear will win, outwitting you.

Aeschylus, 'Agamemnon'[1]

Sobriety did not settle my spirit. After the months working on the home beat passed, I began to feel restless. The dreams and flash-backs of Rwanda had come back. I convinced myself that what was needed was travel to other zones of conflict, to 'put Rwanda in its proper perspective' as I explained to an editor. This was, and I knew it in my heart at the time, an Olympian feat of rationali-sation. I would escape to a different madness, and the unfolding history of the new millennium was about to oblige me.

The century's beginnings provided conflict on a scale that would dwarf the wars of the 1990s. When the attack on the World Trade Center came on 11 September 2001, I was in Colombia reporting on the war between the government and the Marxist guerrillas of FARC – the Revolutionary Armed Forces of Colombia. I watched the Twin Towers blaze and collapse on a television screen in Bogotá and began calling every airline I could to get to New York.

American airspace was shut, so I focused on getting to Pakistan and hopefully crossing the border from there to Afghanistan, where retribution against the Taliban and Al-Qaeda was expected. I agreed with London that I would go to Tajikistan and embed with the forces of the Northern Alliance, who were preparing to march on Kabul and oust the Taliban. American and Allied aircraft were pounding the Taliban and suspected Al-Qaeda bases.

On the evening before I was due to leave, I was struck by fore-boding. A voice in my head told me not to make the trip. Something bad would happen. Never before or since have I had that feeling with such absolute conviction. But how would I explain this to the BBC? I had lobbied to be attached to the invading forces, knowing full well the dangers involved.

The following morning, I was coming down the narrow stairs from the attic room where I usually pack my rucksack before trips. I was wearing socks and I slipped on the carpet. My ankle twisted and I felt a sharp pain. After an X-ray and consultation the doctor told me I had sprained the ligaments in an ankle that had long given me trouble. Rest up for a couple of weeks, he said, then you can go.

I now believe I self-sabotaged. The slip on the stairs was not the accident I pretended to myself at the time. Going down a carpeted stairs in socks carrying a heavy load on my back? At the least, I created the circumstances for a fall.

My presentiment had prevented me from heading to the front. I suspect that my news editor at the BBC understood this, because when I said a few weeks later that I was ready to head out, he asked me if I was sure. 'There is no pressure on you to go.' I was assigned to the theoretically less dangerous refugee story near Quetta, the dusty capital of the Pakistani province of Balochistan, on the border between Pakistan and Afghanistan where, during the Raj, the British had once garrisoned troops to protect against

Afghan attacks. Refugees from the fighting were coming across in their tens of thousands. Among them, it was presumed, were Taliban and Al-Qaeda fighters escaping the American-led assault. It was not really a safe place.

One day at the border we were interviewing a recently arrived family from Kandahar – once the spiritual home of the Taliban and now under relentless air bombardment from the Americans and British. The atmosphere was calm, or appeared so. Then a stone came flying in our direction, then another. Shouting erupted. The disturbance had been started by children and adults who were now gathering. We fled to the car and raced away with volleys of stones flying in our wake.

Many weeks later the journalist Robert Fisk was caught in a similar incident at the same place and badly beaten. His life was saved only by the intercession of an Islamic cleric. Fisk found out afterwards that 'the village housed lots of Afghan refugees, whose relatives had been killed just last week in the American bombing of Kandahar. It doesn't excuse them for beating me up, but there was a real reason why they should hate Westerners.'[2] Fisk's experiences, and our own close shave, showed the dangers of working around angry people. Once the rage of the mob is unleashed it becomes impossible to stop if you are a small group, or a solitary journalist, without protection.

In Quetta there had been suicide blasts in the city and angry crowds demonstrated outside our hotel. We could not leave without a government militia escort. One Saturday morning, as the humanitarian crisis escalated, I made notes back at the hotel:

Translator said war-wounded starting to arrive at the hospital. Staff friendly. Met a man called Nematallah Popolzoi from Kandahar district. Ten-year-son is Said – big dark eyes, was hit by bullet in skull after US bombed a Taliban arms dump. Surgeon says he will live but they can't take bullet out as it is too close to the brain. Impossible to know what prognosis is. Kid in same ward was hit by a car. Looks out of it. Eyes wide open and staring vacantly. Knocked down by a car. So many people are fleeing. Chaos on the roads. Rudimentary facilities here. They need to get him to Islamabad to a skilled neurosurgeon. How likely is that? Met also Nazir Mohammed. Big bandage over his eye. Older men sitting with him. Looks very traumatised. Rocking back and forth. Five-year-old son was killed in the same air strike. Says to me that only someone who has lost a son can understand what he feels. I think about Daniel. He is the same age as that man's kid. There is a grandfather too. He asks me what has his family done to anybody? They never harmed anybody but have lost a grandson. Crying when he said this.

Another day we were invited to meet a group of tribal elders who said they had information on the whereabouts of Osama bin Laden. The meeting took place deep inside the city, down a maze of laneways at the rear of a tailor's shop. The only exit was through the front door. We were invited to sit in a small room at the back. We were three and there were seven of them, younger men than I had expected, but friendly, offering cushions on which to sit and cup after cup of sweet tea. It is an old truism: things in war are often not what they seem to be. Some of the most charming men I have met have also been the most murderous. Every second we spent in that small room I expected kidnappers or assassins to appear. We would only be given the information, they said, if we paid a substantial sum of money. Perhaps our government would be willing to pay?

I took it to be a ruse to try and extort money. We made it clear that we did not represent any government, but politely assured them we would get back with a response from our bosses. As we rose to walk out of shop, I thought: *If they are going to make a move it will be now, before we are out of their grasp.* But we left unmolested.

That night back at the hotel my heart raced – the familiar symptoms of a panic attack, a delayed response to the events of the morning. Now, however, there was no alcoholic oblivion into which I could escape. I recall, in desperation, calling a friend from AA in London. I wanted so badly to pick up a drink. But I was in Pakistan, and not Islamabad or Karachi where waiters had, in the past, found ways to get beer to thirsty journalists. In Quetta at that moment, possessing alcohol could have had extreme consequences. I struggled to speak to my friend through the rapid breathing.

'Paul, I am scared shitless and I need a drink.'

'I understand. Anybody would be. But a drink will just make it worse.'

'How do I get through this fear?'

'Breathe deep. And think of a safe place you know.'

We talked until the waves of panic subsided.

I did what he suggested. I thought of Ardmore in west Waterford and my small tin cottage at the top of Rocky Road, a two-minute walk to the sea, and of the beaches of Curragh and Ballyquin that can be seen from the Storm Wall, our guardian against heavy winter swells, and of evening when music comes through the open window, from the nests of blackbirds and doves in the ruins around the Round Tower. At night, especially in winter when the holiday crowds have gone, you go to sleep to the sound of the sea ebbing and flowing on the bay, and it is joined often by the rattling of the rain on the corrugated roof. I feel truly safe there.

I fell into a half-sleep, the kind that many of my war reporter colleagues will recognise. You doze, but you are still awake – listening for the sound of scuffling feet coming over a wall, or a truck engine approaching the gates. The half-wakefulness is partly because you are scared, and partly because you hope that if they do come that it might add a few seconds to your escape time, or at least ensure you aren't shot or blown to pieces in your sleep.

The war in Afghanistan deposed the Taliban and then dragged on for twenty years. The invasion of Iraq came and I pushed hard to go as a non-embedded reporter, travelling with my own team, not dependent on the military. My old friend from South Africa, Glenn Middleton, the man who filmed the genocide in Rwanda, came with me.

I remember clinging to the pavement on the banks of the Tigris in Baghdad, as US Marines unloaded volley after volley of automatic fire at snipers on the other side of the river: press the trigger, blaze away, load again, repeat, until a voice can make itself heard shouting 'cease fire' to young men high on exhaustion and adrenaline. Baghdad in the days of invasion, 2003: the helicopter gunships and the fighter planes; twilights of black smoke against a red sun, an old man scouring the freshly dug graves in the hospital garden looking for his missing son, medical equipment looted from clinics by the mob. More adrenaline, sleepless nights camped out on a flint-hard desert, nights in abandoned buildings, once even in Saddam Hussein's palace in his hometown of Tikrit.

That war killed other people I knew: Terry Lloyd of ITN, shot dead with cameraman Frédéric Nérac and their Iraqi translator Hussein Osman on 22 March. Eight days later, Gaby Rado of Channel 4 News fell to his death from the roof of a hotel in northern Iraq. A few days after that, cameraman Kaveh Golestan was killed and my friend Stuart Hughes lost a leg when they stepped on landmines in Kifri in the north. Then came a 'friendly fire' air strike by the Americans on 6 April which killed an Iraqi colleague, Kamran Abdulrazaq Mohammed, and left my dear friend Fred Scott and colleague John Simpson wounded. It happened while they were travelling with a Kurdish force.

For all the triumphalism that followed the fall of Saddam's statue it smelt like a war that was only starting. On the way back from Tikrit we saw Marine gunships come down the river all roar and power as they skimmed low; a young man on the street turned towards us and drew his finger across his throat. I saw Abrams tanks unleashing their awful firepower towards villages, and in the hospital at al-Hilla counted the child victims of allied cluster munitions.

When I was asked to go back to Iraq during the insurgency that followed Saddam's fall, I refused. In a newspaper interview around this time, I said I would not cover any more 'hot wars' – in other words I would go to the aftermaths of conflicts only, or to the refugee crises that drive people across international borders seeking safety. This is how I described my decision in 2005:

So I made myself a new rule: I would try to avoid places where bullets were flying. And would make far fewer trips. Shouldn't I have done that years ago? Of course. But my adult life has been about finding the courage to change. It takes time but I am getting there … I am not always calm or serene; I am not 'resolved' or 'redeemed'. I am still prey to sad moods, flashes of anger, dissatisfactions I cannot assuage or understand. Perhaps the change is that I am learning to live with it.[3]

I wince now when I read those words. I see the repeating pattern. I did make fewer trips. I invested in the lives of my children with time and love. But I still went to the wars. And I was not 'learning to live' with the trauma of war. The warning signs kept flashing.

In Qana of the Miracles I smelt wild lavender
All the way down a country lane,
Where a dead child in Mickey Mouse pyjamas
Was carried from the rubble, stiffening
Into dead weight in the arms of his father
Whose eyes were closed,
As if he was carrying his boy to bed.
I wished you had been beside me, Michael.
For you alone could tell this
With the tenderness it deserved.
That night I fell asleep with diazepam,
And a copy of *Snow Water*.
Awoken by artillery after four,
I was still clutching your book.
The windows shook and I held tight to your words.
I am grateful to you my friend,
For the fragments of sanity you send.[4]

On the way back to Tyre my fear of an Israeli drone strike has given way to a deep exhaustion. I have the sensation of floating high above the chalky hills between Qana and the coast, out over where Hezbollah fires its rockets at Israeli civilians and past the Israeli gunboats nestling in the aquamarine of the Mediterranean. The mind is doing what the body cannot. I am grateful. In the language of PTSD, this is called dissociation – where a protective psyche puts distance between us and the trauma we are witnessing. It is an old defence of mine.

Within a year of writing that I was going to avoid 'hot wars', I was in south Lebanon covering the conflict between the Israelis and Hezbollah.

The poem above is my own, found in a file while I was compulsively sorting and resorting scraps of memories in the middle of a mental breakdown. I looked for notes made on the road in one messed-up country or another. I thought that some pattern might emerge, a tentative map of where my mind had travelled in the years of observing the suffering of others. I wrote the poem in honour of a friend and great poet, Michael Longley, whose work had been a consolation through many wars, and which I first read in Belfast, during my early days of reporting conflict.

I turned to Michael after the Qana airstrike. *All of these people, alive or dead are civilised.*[5] The strike took place on 30 July 2006 and was the first and only time I broke down on air, although background noise prevented the audience from guessing what had happened. Twenty-eight people were killed, sixteen of them children. The basement in which they'd been sleeping became a tomb when the house was struck by a huge Israeli bomb.* I was being

---

* The Israeli Defence Force later said that it had attacked the building without knowing there were civilians inside. The IDF said Hezbollah had fired rockets towards Israel from the area and used civilians as human shields. Amnesty International and Human Rights Watch criticised the IDF's explanation and demanded an independent inquiry.

interviewed on the BBC when I saw the men of the village carrying some of the dead children out of the house. Most of those I saw showed no outward sign of injury. The bomb had efficiently sucked the oxygen out of the basement and suffocated them, leaving them covered by a thick film of dust. Inside the little bodies, vital organs had been turned into a mulch by the blast wave. But they did not appear dead, not immediately. Then the wailing of the mothers started up.

The dead at Qana were not the first child corpses I had seen in war, but there was something about the domesticity of the scene, the broken tenderness in the face of a father cradling his dead son, that made me falter in my live interview.

There were essential truths that television news could try to communicate – the who, how and why of what happened, some of the grief and pain – and then there were individual lifetimes of loss that could never be conveyed. I knew that nothing I could tell of this would make the slightest difference in the long run. The war might end here in south Lebanon but somewhere else in the world, adults would go on fighting with the inevitable consequence that children would die.

In the previous few days, I had been part of a convoy that came under attack from Israeli mortars on the road between the Christian village of Rmeish, about a mile from the Israeli border, and the coastal city of Tyre, where the international media was based. We travelled during a temporary halt in the fighting, but along the way passed vehicles that had been hit by Israeli strikes, a reminder of the constant danger along this route. The village was packed with Shiite Muslim refugees who may have believed that Rmeish, being Christian, and not a Hezbollah stronghold, would be less of a target for the Israelis. In the basement of Tajali Maronite church they pressed around us, pleading to be taken out of the front line in our small convoy. They were without a proper water supply and children were already becoming ill.

We set off back along the coast road, refugee vehicles interspersed among our own, and prayed the ceasefire would hold. I cannot remember how long it took but I vividly recall the first shell landing in front of us, a cloud of black smoke erupting from the roadside. Our driver and bodyguard, a former member of the British special forces, accelerated and within seconds we were passing a car that had been hit.

I do not remember any debate. Instinct kicked in. We stopped. I jumped out with a colleague and raced back to the stricken vehicle. At any second I expected more mortars. Two men sat inside the car, both were wounded. At that moment I could not tell how seriously. As we got closer I could see the man nearest to me in the driver's seat was bleeding from the neck, but the rest of his body was intact. We opened the doors and reached in to help them out. My man would not move: he sat staring straight ahead. Then he said he did not want to leave the car. It was his car, even if it had been shot up by shrapnel. It might be stolen if he left it.

I shouted something like: 'You can stay here and fucking die or you can come with me and live.' I reached in again and he put his arm around my neck and allowed himself to be half-walked, half-dragged to our vehicle. Once inside I cleaned the wound in his neck and patched him. His face was grey with terror. We were dependent now on the decisions and mathematical calculations of the Israeli mortar teams. Would they be told to fire again, and if they were, could rapid speed evade the arc of their shells? We drove furiously until the road turned away from the direct line of sight of the Israelis and towards a UN base, where an Irish colonel opened the gates and took the wounded man and his colleague to a field hospital.

Nobody spoke on the journey back to Tyre. On the way down to Rmeish that morning I had memorised certain landmarks – a ruined bridge we'd driven around onto the dried riverbed, a truck mangled by a missile, an overgrown olive plantation. It was a way of keeping my mind off the Israeli drones overhead. The landmarks now became my waystations on the drive to safety, each one ticked off as we came closer to the city. We kept the windows down, listening for the whine of drones above us and knew that if one were fired, we would be dead before we even heard the explosion. When we pulled into the hotel a colleague came up to greet us. 'You need to wash your hands, mate,' he said. I looked and saw that they were covered in the dried blood of the injured man. A friend from ITN came over to check how I was. They hadn't been on our convoy. He made a joke: 'A good result all round. Light injuries and great TV.' I could take that. There was a cynical truth in what he said, even if it was prompted by envy at missing out on the story. I would be praised for the power of the piece that night. The bosses would note the team's bravery. All's well that ends well. Until it doesn't.

In Tyre I had already seen a person smashed into the air by the impact of an ambulance racing to rescue the wounded in the hills outside the city. I saw people staggering from a bombed building, weaving around me in shock amid billowing dust and smoke. On the day of an evacuation at the harbour, I ran along the pier with colleagues, carrying in our arms some of the children of a Palestinian family, but we only managed to get the mother and a daughter to the boats on time. Her young sons missed evacuation by minutes. The mother waved frantically from the rowing boat that was heading to the ship lying offshore. There was nothing to be done. The boys were left behind in a refugee camp with their father. I visited them a few days later to see how they were holding up, if there had been any news from his wife. The father was friendly – yes, she had been in touch and was on her way to Denmark but it didn't look like there would be another evacuation for a long time.

Then a ceasefire came. It usually does when the level of slaughter gets too embarrassing for the international community. The Red Crescent and various NGOs began clearing up the rubble. Some of the unexploded bombs were removed. Others remained. Bodies were found and buried. I left for holidays. Then I went back to an older war.

I did this. Then I did that. I went here. After that I went there. And there too. I saw this and that, and then more and more. But does it mean anything at this stage of the story? By now have you not had proof enough of the state of my reckless, addicted mind? Christ, I am weary writing this, thinking about what it says of who I was in those days. But that is the point: clarity only emerges for me as I set this down. Not every place told an easily defined story of psychological disintegration, but they would accumulate and set my face towards a reckoning.

There are repeat trips to the Democratic Republic of Congo: I see ransacked houses by the side of the road, an ambushed vehicle, a mortuary with no working lights where we view the dead of a massacre by the light of dusk, a vehicle in our convoy broken down in the middle of the night, guarded by nervous soldiers who know that rebels can come from anywhere; I see Vulumilia Lakando, a sixteen-year-old girl from a village above Goma, who was gang-raped by so many militia that she passed out, and who is now incontinent, the urine dripping onto the earth as she stands; I meet the 'Protestant Women of Kachenga', who care for the rape victims, and the doctors in Goma and Bukavu, whose skill and gentleness allow hope to flicker; I see a night by Lake Kivu when the lightning leaps and for a few moments I forget the cruelties to which innocent people are subjected.

I eventually give up going to Congo because I am threatened by the supporters of a Tutsi warlord who is busy terrorising and looting and believes he should be allowed to carry on without suffering the prying eyes of foreign reporters.

I am not drinking, but for all the talk about not covering hot wars anymore I am taking bigger risks than ever. I go to places where there is no protection to be had from the authorities. I know the dangers, but my need to be there overwhelms reason.

Fred Scott and I go to Darfur, where the government of Sudan has instigated a genocide against African tribes that will kill up to 400,000 people and displace millions more. Mass rape accompanies this first genocide of the twenty-first century. One night we decide to stay in a refugee camp, where residents fearfully await a raid by the security forces. We have spent the afternoon interviewing people who tell of their sufferings at the hands of the police and the 'Janjaweed', the so-called 'devils on horseback', who carry out the worst of the atrocities.

For weeks the police have been trying to deport the residents away from the town and deeper into the desert, where UN officials in the area will find it harder to monitor their welfare. My rationale is that in order to show to the world what is happening, we have to be present when these raids take place.

There is no possibility of sleeping, not with the certainty that a raid is coming. In the early hours we hear vehicles approaching and see headlights tracking through the camp. We are told to hide. A man rushes us into a mud hut where rice is stored. I hear the sounds of blows, of shacks being knocked over by pickup trucks, of people being assaulted. Women are screaming.

Fred asks: 'What the fuck do we do if they find us?'

'We hope they don't shoot before asking questions,' I reply.

It is not bravado. I am terrified but believe if we have the time to say who we are and show our BBC ID there is a good chance we will come out of this safely.

The militia do not discover our hiding place, but the following morning they return. Tear gas is fired at crowds of women and children queuing outside an aid clinic. They scatter in the panic; small children stumble and fall over and vomit from the effects of the gas. Sticks smash again into bodies already weakened by hunger. The police spot Fred filming and fire a plastic bullet directly at us. It misses by inches. A UN worker says that we should go before the cops arrest us. We run towards the roadway, through a maze of shacks, until we reach a vehicle and drive fast into town.

Fred and I have an angry row. I don't remember what sparked it, but at its root was fear. There have, for both of us, been too many close shaves in bad places recently. It was just a year since Fred was almost killed by US friendly fire in Iraq.

Word comes that the police are looking for us. We are over a thousand kilometres from the capital, in a town where the security forces run the show. We don't want to fall into their hands, so we call a colleague in Khartoum who charters a plane to come and collect us. The idea is that we will get to Khartoum to catch a flight out to London that night, something we hope the Sudanese are not anticipating. The local airport is deserted apart from a few porters and someone in the control tower. I keep expecting the police to arrive and haul us away. Then I hear the engines of a jet. Our transport is a hulking machine that has seen better days; the rear cargo door does not close properly. The choice is wait and be arrested or get out on this plane and trust it makes it to the other end.

We make it in time to catch a flight to London. Nobody stops us at immigration and our tapes safely make it through customs.

We are out. First comes the relief, after that the low – the going home, the struggle to become a husband and father who can engage in daily life. And I think about the row with Fred: two already traumatised people snapping under the strain. He says to me later that he wonders if our presence hadn't made things worse for the people in the camp. The police had spotted us filming the evening before. Maybe the night raid on the camp was punishment for the displaced cooperating with us? I didn't know one way or the other. But that question unsettles me. As a journalist if you cannot make things better, you at least should not make things worse.

I promise – again – to try not to go to hot wars. I try, but in a typically disingenuous way. Rather than go to the shooting and bombing, I focus more on undercover reporting, on human rights abuses in Myanmar, and then Zimbabwe.

This brings a different kind of stress than the existential terror of death by sniper, bomb or machete. Once you have crossed the border into a state where there is no rule of law, pretending to be somebody you are not – in my case a tourist, or businessman rather than a journalist – all bets are potentially off. At the least you could expect a beating and temporary incarceration in a dreadful prison before, hopefully, being deported. At worst you might get the beating and a long prison sentence or be disappeared.

I had been travelling to Myanmar since the first release from house arrest in 1995 of Aung San Suu Kyi, then the icon of the pro-democracy movement, her future as the denier of ethnic cleansing and genocide in Rakhine State impossible to imagine then. I formed a personal bond with her. I was flattered that I was the first foreign correspondent allowed to interview her after her release, and that she had listened to my broadcasts while confined. I believed her when she spoke in the language of Gandhi and Martin Luther King, and when she praised Nelson Mandela as an inspiration.

For me, and for much of the world, Aung San Suu Kyi was the antidote to Milošević in the Balkans, or the Hutu extremists in Rwanda – a woman who spoke the language of universal human rights, and whose charisma became a screen onto which journalists, diplomats, human rights workers, and her own supporters, projected their hopes. She seemed to be everything a genocide-haunted reporter could want her to be.

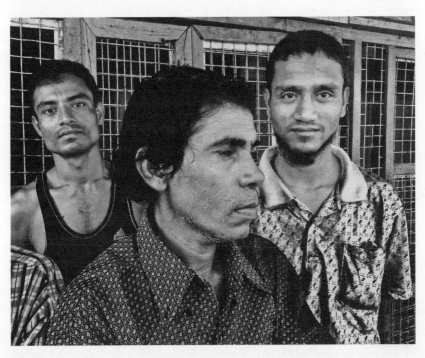

A scene from Myanmar in an era of upheaval.

In August 2007 protests erupted against price rises caused by the regime's withdrawal of fuel subsidies. Buddhist Monks assumed a prominent role, leading journalists to describe the demonstrations as the 'Saffron Revolution', after the colour of the monks' robes. I felt nervous about going there. I was now on a regime blacklist. They would be watching out for journalists they regarded as enemies. In the past, with the benefits of dual-nationality I had been able to juggle passports in a way that managed to confuse the people at passport control. Astonishingly tourists were still being allowed into the country, despite the fact of the demonstrations, the murder of monks and activists and the arrests of thousands.

Eyewitnesses described pitiless attacks: 'Some people in the crowd were killed. They shot three people in the foreheads and their skulls exploded in the back, one of them was hit in the temple. These three were middle-aged persons. One child was shot in the chest [and died].'[6]

The night before I am due to leave for Yangon, the nerve-twisting anxieties begin. I know the junta's security apparatus has spies everywhere; there will be the constant threat of being caught.

By the time I am in the queue for passport control the following day I am in full panic mode. *Will they recognise me from BBC World TV? Have they been tipped off in advance by the embassy in Bangkok? … Johnny from Channel 4 said they have photographs of the hacks they hate posted inside the immigration booths. Maybe they will let me in and then tail me until they can arrest me along with the interviewees … Remember how they beat up our cameraman Darren and kicked him out. Still, at least they didn't find any of his tapes – a good result for him, all things considered.*

I struggle to control my heart rate. *Breathe deep. Look the immigration officer in the eyes, smile.*

He calls his superior over. The two of them scrutinise my documents and then my face. Still smiling. Some words I don't understand. My passport is stamped, and I am nodded in. I cannot let my guard down: between immigration and customs is perhaps fifty yards, and here spooks from military intelligence loiter, face-checking arriving Westerners. I get through, look in the taxi driver's mirror to make sure I am not being shadowed and head into town.

Daily undercover operating involves discipline. I have a set of rules which I hope will keep me from discovery and arrest:

Keep your story simple. Make sure the cover is a story you
    start to believe yourself.
Say nothing on the phone that doesn't sound like tourist
    blather.
Schedule several tourist activities each day so that anybody
    watching won't be suspicious.
Never leave a compromising document/piece of paper in your
    hotel room.
Destroy all notes when you're finished with them.
Change taxis at least twice on your way to and from
    appointments with dissident figures. Lose yourself in
    markets and busy public places if you suspect you are being
    followed.
Never identify an informant on camera. Film the back of their
    heads or in silhouette – talking to the foreign media could
    get them tortured or even killed.
Never travel with your tapes. Find an alternative route for
    them out of the country.

I assume the police are watching my hotel and so make no plans to meet any of the protestors or dissidents there. I walk around the city, ostentatiously displaying my Lonely Planet Guide to Burma. Surely it occurs to these malign bastards that tourists with any sense have cancelled their holidays in the middle of the bloodletting?

The only way I can meet with the monks who are in hiding is to leave the hotel before the curfew lifts at first light. The Thai producer, Annie, accompanies me. We try to play the role of a couple who just happen to be going out before curfew to see the dawn rise. I offer to pay the taxi driver double his fee and he agrees, saying that he knows roads where there are no military checkpoints. Of course it occurs to us that he may be working for the military, and what then? We drive out in the dark. Every car light I see coming sets my heart pounding. This is not work for a mind that deep down is starting to fracture. Yet, I reason, I have come all this way to get the story. This journey is unavoidable.

I make it to the meeting point without being stopped by the secret police. The cameraman, who is also Thai, arrives separately. He is less conspicuous here. I interview the monks in a small room above a shop. I am conscious of every minute that passes. I talk to them about their experiences of the regime for around half an hour. When I am satisfied that we have not been tailed, and the hiding place is still secure, I follow a circuitous route through backstreets and through a church compound until I find a taxi.

That evening, back at the hotel, I run into an old friend from my days living in Hong Kong. She tells me that I look strange. 'I've never seen you look so stressed,' she says. 'Are you okay?' Was I okay? No, not at all. But I tell her everything is fine. Just the pressure of deadlines.

The journey out of Myanmar is nerve-shredding. The same suspicious stares. The unnatural silence of a departure lounge where the plain-clothes government men mingle among the passengers and those of us who are not who we say we are – I am sure I am not alone – wait for the fateful approach. I make it through, but even as the plane takes off, I am still not right. The 'buzz' I've become used to getting from this has gone. I don't feel hyper alive with adrenaline in the old way. Just desperate. Shit scared.

Once home, I am constantly tired but struggle to sleep at night. I battle on with nightmares. My anxiety and depression are deepening. I fixate on just about anything now. Only in the afternoons, while it is still light and feels safe, can I sleep. The only cure is going out on the road again, which is no cure at all.

13

Old Ground

> Can the few who survived these horrors ever really recover? …
> I do not know, for, though I have spent weeks in this blighted
> country, I cannot imagine what such suffering must do to the
> minds and hearts of human beings.
>
> David Orr, journalist, letter to Raymond Mbaraga, Rwanda
> genocide survivor, 16 February 2021[1]

I would not call this visitation a nightmare. There was no fear
attached to the experience. The girl sat at the end of my bed. My
mouth moved to ask who she was, but no words came. Nor did
she speak. That is how we remained, in the suspended time of a
dream, for how long I cannot say, until I woke and found that I
was full of sadness, and morning was still hours away.

It was Rwanda that eventually brought the house crashing
down. It happened in 2008, fourteen years after the genocide
occurred. The breakdown I experienced took me away from work
for the best part of a year. It was also the beginning of the first
conscious effort to deal with my PTSD.

The surprise is that the crash took so long. After leaving
Butare in June 1994 we came home, made our film, and moved

on to our different lives. The documentary was watched by a small audience. There was one newspaper review. By then the genocide had been overtaken by news of hundreds of thousands of Hutu refugees fleeing into Zaire, among them many of the perpetrators of the slaughter. The French sent troops to create so called 'safe zones', an act that rescued some Tutsis but allowed many of France's old friends in the Hutu extremist ranks to escape.

I went to Vancouver to the wedding of my sister. The nightmares began there and continued after I came back. In the most frequent I would dream myself under a pile of corpses with a machete-wielding killer trying to find me. Then there was the apparition of the silent girl at the end of my bed.

The following year I won prizes for reporting on the genocide. I felt guilty that I was acclaimed. But not enough to reject the awards. I needed them. They were my substitute for self-worth. In her essay *Regarding the Pain of Others* Susan Sontag writes of those 'star witnesses, renowned for their bravery and zeal', but whose reports 'nourish belief in the inevitability of tragedy in the benighted or backward – that is, poor – parts of the world'.[2] I flinched reading that. I had always told myself that I aimed at a journalism that would set Rwanda in the context of a universal understanding of genocide, an impulse that could grow in the hearts of people *everywhere*, given a specific set of circumstances.

Yet I worked in a medium that depended on imagery for its storytelling power, and those pictures of Africans with machetes and clubs, and mounds of bodies, inevitably had the effect described by Susan Sontag. The dead were not only stripped of their humanity by the killers, reduced to bones and rotting flesh; they were trapped there by our images. The cameras could not record the lives, lives the dead had lived – working, loving, lust-ing, raising children, dreaming, the lives of people who went to school, looked at the night sky, swam in the fast streams of the rainy season, walked cattle through the grasslands on the Tanzanian border, those who looked once upon 'the colour of nostalgia, the mauve of the Jacaranda trees' in Butare.[3]

Moral injury came not only from the feeling of failing as a human being, but from disillusionment with the whole journalistic enterprise. I am conscious that my experience cannot begin to compare to those who survived genocide. I was only a witness to parts of what had happened. My time in the country was counted in weeks, not the three months of relentless horror, and I had a ticket out, the return to a safe place. In the years afterwards I regularly met with survivors who saw their loved ones murdered, as well as the victims of gang rape and mutilation by drunken mobs of militiamen and opportunist criminals. As Rwanda struggled to create a stable society, genocide survivors found themselves living next to the people who killed their families, many of them released from prison under a reconciliation process known as Gacaca.*

Rates of PTSD were soaring. Among one group of survivors, psychologists found a suicide rate of 25 per cent. Trauma was also infecting the lives of foreign witnesses, like the UN officers and staff of the International Committee of the Red Cross who stayed in Rwanda through the entire hundred days of killing. Captain Stefan Stec, a Polish UN officer, risked his life trying to save besieged Tutsi communities and years later, in 2005, was reportedly harangued for the UN's failures at a showing of the film

---

* The Gacaca system saw those accused of genocide at a 'lower level' – the peasants who killed their neighbours – called before village meetings where they were asked to confess their crimes in return for the possibility of a lighter jail sentence.

Hotel Rwanda in the Hague. Afterwards he stopped eating until his body eventually gave out and he died that same year. Stec's death was described in a newspaper as having come about 'in spite of help from psychiatrists who had treated soldiers from the Dutch battalion in Srebrenica ...'[4]

A sense of guilt led me into a preoccupation with genocide. I made films on the Armenians, Darfur and the Holocaust. I went back to the Rwandan story repeatedly, after I knew it was inflicting further damage on my mental health. I believed there was a chance that with the creation of international tribunals, and building a political will to intervene, genocide might be prevented. To do this, memory needed to be refreshed constantly. It was necessary too to comprehend, not to indulge what one aid agency chief reasonably called 'compassion without understanding'. I also needed to appreciate what had happened in the minds of those who killed: what created the circumstances in which a human being would kill their neighbour? There was a selfish element to this investigation. If I could apply the light of rational calculation to the stuff of my nightmares, there was a possibility they would end. I might also – this is what I believed then, I stress – affect the policy of governments that wanted to look the other way. It was never my conscious intention to re-traumatise myself.

Ten years after the genocide, I went back to meet the men and women who had hacked and clubbed their fellow citizens at road-blocks, carried out massacres in churches at the urging of the local mayors, entered into their neighbour's houses and hunted them down in banana groves and swamps. Some were still in prison, others had served their sentences. Such was the extent of mass participation in violence, Rwanda could never have held all of the killers in lifetime detention.

To prepare myself, I re-read transcripts of interviews I had made during the genocide. I sought out some of the words broadcast by the extremist Radio des Mille Collines ('Radio of the Thousand Hills') played on transistor radios at roadblocks, in military bases, and in the homes of the leaders of the massacres. I had heard it in the refugee camps to which Hutu perpetrators fled to escape the invading Tutsi army: 'The day when the people rise up and want no more of you, when they hate you all together and from the bottom of their hearts, when you make them sick to their stomachs, I wonder then where will you escape to, where will you go …?'[5]

Some of those I interviewed were defensive, careful about what they would admit to. Post-genocide Rwanda was still a fearful place in which those on the losing side made wary calculations about how much and what kind of truth or lie the victors and the victims should hear. Yet the level of frankness in our day-to-day encounters surprised me.

For some of the perpetrators there was also great trauma to be reckoned with. They had killed, raped and looted like people gone mad. Blood spurted, formed pools on floors and flowed into gutters. Ravening dogs trotted in the wake of the death squads. Clouds of carrion hunters alighted from the roofs and trees. Nothing in the anatomy of man or woman was hidden to the children who saw parents chop their neighbours down. In other times, in different circumstances, most of the killers would never have acted in this way. But they lived in a place and time where killing was declared by the state to be as natural as eating or drinking and was, moreover, a patriotic obligation. Hate, envy, spite, greed, lust – all were given permission to riot across the hills without limits. Some peasants were told that if they did not kill the Tutsi, they themselves would be killed.

'Hate can be reassuring and self-protective,' one study declared, 'because its message is simple and helps confirming people's belief in a just world.'[6] Justice was to be achieved with the destruction of the Tutsi enemy. The category of enemy brooked no exceptions: armed combatants and civilians, men, women, children; the young and the old.

Besides the sheer scale of the slaughter, the inversion of the moral order made Rwanda psychologically devastating: I was confronted with a society mobilised for a campaign of murder that was the personal duty of every patriotic citizen. There was no possibility in Rwanda of looking the other way, as millions of Germans had once done, at least those far enough from the chimneys of the death camps, or the railway stations of deportation. Broken windows, the beating of Jews in the streets, vile anti-Semitic propaganda – these were stations along the way to mass murder, but the final act was witnessed by comparatively few citizens of the Reich. In Rwanda the killing was impossible to avoid.

It is possible that many of those I met on my return would have been happy to see the end of Rwanda's new Tutsi-dominated government. Some might have wished to finish the job of exterminating the minority. But for a genocide defendant to express such a sentiment would have made a bad predicament much, much worse. Nearly all blamed either the former Hutu government, or Satan, for leading them to kill. 'Why else would you start butchering your neighbour?' one asked me. The resort to a metaphysical answer was not wholly self-serving. Just as my forebears had told ghost stories to mediate the experience of mass death in the Great Hunger, here rural communities, steeped in the Catholic faith but also in ancestral folk traditions, might seek to explain the violence through the prism of evil and irresistible forces. Yet rationalisations could not protect the mind entirely from guilt for the horrors they had perpetrated. Many were obviously struggling with their memories.

During the genocide in 1994, I walked through the aftermath of the massacre at Nyarubuye, a parish in south-western Rwanda close to the Tanzanian border. The place reeked of the corpses that lay in the church grounds, the diocesan offices, the mission school, between the rows of seats in the church itself, and on the front steps beneath a falling banner proclaiming the feast of Christ's Resurrection. There were different estimates of the dead – from hundreds to more than 20,000. They would still be unearthing corpses as late as 2012, when the bodies of several women, thought to have been raped, were found buried in newly excavated latrines. Walking into that place, I felt mentally detached from the horror, as if I was moving on autopilot. Darkness fell. We left the main scene of slaughter and, as we walked, our torches glanced on a desiccated corpse here, a few scraps of flesh and bone there. We kept the beams pointing directly in front of our feet, until we could be sure of walking without trampling on the remains of the slain.

One of the leaders of the massacre told me later: 'When we moved in, it was as if we were competing over the killing. We entered and each one of us began killing their own. When we were walking into the classrooms we were wearing rubber boots because of all the blood. There was so much blood that it was flowing like a river.'[7]

Evariste Maherane killed at Nyarubuye. He was a free man when I met him, after serving six years in prison, and was living with his wife and children and grandson. He remembered during the genocide hearing about a Tutsi boy who escaped the church where his parents had been killed. The child was about ten years old. A local Hutu family had taken him in. When Evariste and another killer arrived at the Hutu house they demanded that the boy be handed over. Dressed in his school-issue khaki shorts and shirt, the boy had been wounded in the attack which killed his parents. Though he'd been given some medicine by the Hutu family he was weak. Evariste took the child and marched him into a banana plantation. Evariste held him by the neck and battered him with a club. The other killer joined in. Then they dug a hole, and pushed him in.

'Was he still alive when you buried him?' I asked.

'Yes, he was still alive.'

Evariste had a ten-year-old son of his own at the time of the killing. He said that he was haunted by the memory of the Tutsi child's arms and legs flailing in the smothering earth. 'It was a time of hatred. Our heads were hot. We were animals.'[8] The picture of the dying boy shifting under the earth would never leave him.

There was Silas Ngendahimana who, had I met him on a roadblock in 1994, would have terrified me. Six feet tall, with a powerful physique and intensely staring eyes, he remembered the moment he first set out to kill. 'I had thought about the plan overnight. I woke up, washed my face and left. I felt no pain or sorrow … because the government had given up on them, I went to kill without tears. I went to kill feeling well. I went and did what I had come to do, to kill.'[9]

Silas was searching for food in the convent adjacent to the church when he heard someone breathing under a bed. He looked underneath and saw a terrified woman. He dragged her out.

'Did she ask you for mercy,' I asked him.

'Yes, she did, but you have to understand mercy wasn't part of the deal. The government had given them up to us to be killed.'

'But you didn't have to kill her,' I said. 'You were alone with her in the room. You could have left her hiding there. That wasn't the government's fault.'

Silas explained calmly that if he had allowed the woman to live, she might have reported him for stealing property. So, he beat her with his nail-studded club until her screaming stopped. Then he continued his search for food and found a bag of meal.[10]

Before leaving the area he looked around. 'There was a water tap that was running and mixing with the blood,' he remembers. 'We could only step in the small spaces that had not been stained in order to leave that place.'[11]

Silas killed because others were killing, because those were his orders, because there were spoils to be reaped from the looting of his neighbours. But he was visibly disturbed now by the memory of the woman pleading, the blood on the ground.

Most atrocities are not committed by psychopaths. There simply would not have been enough of them to carry out the kind of killing that happened in Rwanda, or in the Holocaust, or the Armenian genocide, or any of the more recent mass slaughters. It is the horror that is perpetrated by people with no psychiatric disorder, the potential of the monster within us all, that was exposed in my long conversations with the Rwandan killers.

I addressed my desire to understand. But I did not learn to accept. Not the hatred that had infected so many, or the guilt that lingered inside me. I tried to assuage it with continued reporting about the genocide and involvement in charity. I also agreed to testify in the Rwandan genocide trials taking place in the Tanzanian city of Arusha under the auspices of the UN. I testified once for the prosecution, and once for the defence, my rationale being that in a courtroom, where I answered questions from both sides, justice would be served, and I would add my tiny portion to the institutional memory of the genocide. I did not reckon then with the potential mental health consequences of testifying.

The first trial involved only a morning in the witness box, testifying in the trial of the leader of the massacre at Nyarubuye. As I had not been present during the slaughter, there was only a limited amount of information I could bring to the proceedings.

The Butare trial in October 2006 was of a different order. Widely regarded as one of the most significant of the genocide cases, it involved the prosecution of several government ministers and senior officials, and some of the most horrific testimony to be placed before the International Criminal Tribunal for Rwanda. I had been present, with my colleagues, for a short period during the actual killings in Butare, and I had travelled with the convoy of Tutsi orphans to the border. I was called to testify by the defence for the former *préfet*, Sylvain Nsabimana. My testimony would not be decisive. I would describe what I saw, nothing else. But I was independent in the eyes of both the defence and prosecution. I felt I owed it to the dead.

14

Trials

... yet from those flames
No light; but rather darkness visible
Served only to discover sights of woe ...

Paradise Lost, John Milton[1]

I felt alone and needed help. I had arrived in Arusha the previous day, to a city filled with sunlight, and walked the jacaranda-lined streets as if I were one of the tourists thronging here on their way to and from the national parks and Mount Kilimanjaro. This Arusha was the Africa of the Western imagination, a post-colonial fantasy of 'charming natives' and gorgeous sights, the opposite of the other trope, which Rwanda represented, of endless massacre and irrational hatreds.

I had come here as a witness and wondered if my fellow Westerners were aware of the other stories being told in the UN courtroom in this city? I could not have felt more detached from the happy faces with their bush khaki and floppy hats and Lonely Planet guides. I went back to my room, trying to remember, trying to forget, my anxiety growing at the prospect of the week to come. The night before I was due in court, I wrote to my editor:

198

I am in Arusha and take the stand tomorrow. It has now transpired that I am to be questioned by Nsabimana's attorney, then cross-examined by five other attorneys for the other defendants in the case and also the prosecution. That means seven cross examinations in all. Jon, I am already feeling very wobbly and struggle to sleep. I feel a huge sense of being alone here with the memory of that time bearing down on me ...

I met with Nsabimana's counsel, Josette Kadji, a clever young woman from Cameroon who did her best to make me feel at ease. It was impossible. We went through the procedures for the morning. I told her that I felt apprehensive facing people I had not seen since the genocide, but I did not speak of trauma. I wanted to be a steady witness. In my messages to London, however, I describe spending the morning looking at 'old rushes' (tapes we filmed in 1994) with Nsabimana's defence. 'By the end of it I could hardly speak. I dread the next few days.'

There was no sleep that night. I lay awake repeating my mantra: *Only say what you can remember. Do not offer opinions. No rising to any provocation by a counsel. Look directly at the judges. Speak slowly and carefully. Take as much time as you need to respond.*

I was collected by the UN police in the morning. The city passed me by in a blur of cars and human figures. Then I was immersed in the bureaucracy of the court. There were forms to fill in. A last meeting with Josette. 'I hope you are not too nervous,' she smiled.

I was sick to my stomach, but I just nodded.

As I sat down in the witness box, I saw Sylvain Nsabimana sitting directly opposite. He did not look to have aged very much. We looked at each other. I did not smile. I cannot now remember if he did. The panel of three judges sat directly ahead of me, and to the left, along with their counsel and the other defendants, Pauline Nyiramasuhuko and Shalom Ntahobali.

This is where it ended – the trail of blood, bits of brain and bowel, the body waste of refugees, of rapists' semen, the cologne of the murder bosses, the sweat of the killers and their victims, all of that now to be remembered in a place that was odourless and sterile.

I sat there, hour after hour, over several days while lawyers in long black gowns called me back to the events of that murderous summer, every eye in that courtroom focused on me. Excerpts of our footage were played: images from a hospital where we filmed as shells landed outside – a child with his arm hacked off, a woman screaming 'My God, My God ...'

I was back there – crossing the militia checkpoints to get to the hospital and back again to the rebel side; the militia staring, sitting at street corners, red-eyed and drunk; crossing the valley between the two armies by Land Rover, praying to Christ above there would be no mortars like the ones that killed a Senegalese peacekeeper on this same route.

I broke down and had to leave the box. I was shaking and dry heaving in the toilet adjacent to the court.

There are moments when the kindness of others can break a spell. I will always cherish the tenderness shown by two Tanzanian men who worked for the court, John Kiyeyeu and Emmanuel Mwanja. They accompanied me to the bathroom and showed me that I was not alone. 'Take your time,' they said. 'Be calm.' 'Would you like some water?' 'We will only go back when you are ready ...'

I called the BBC in London and asked them to send somebody to support me. The official policy is that any decision to testify is personal. But I have never been refused help when I've asked for it. An old friend from South Africa, Milton Nkosi, my producer and best friend during the township wars, flew up from Johannesburg. He arrived at the hotel smiling and held me in a powerful embrace. After that when I got into the box, I was conscious of Milton sitting behind me, beyond the glass screen that separated the trial chamber from the body of the court. I felt his strength. I got through.

Before leaving for home, I wrote to my editor. A full twelve years after the genocide, I was at last asking for specific psychological help for the first time.

I am writing because I think I will need access to post-traumatic stress counselling when I get back. I would be very grateful if the BBC could recommend somebody who specialises in war trauma. I did not expect to feel so overwhelmed ...

Fergal

I know that somebody from management called me. I was given a phone number for an assessment. But I never followed it up. Instead, I returned to the places of pain. I suspect it makes no sense to you. But I am in the grip of a compulsion more powerful even than my addiction to alcohol.

By the late winter of 2008 my nightmares were back with force. I dreamed vividly of the dead, horrible images that caused me to wake sweating, sometimes fighting in my sleep with arms flailing, knocking over my bedside lamp. I had experienced such symptoms immediately after the genocide but now they were accompanied by crippling anxiety. Panic attacks kept me in bed for days. I stopped shaving and only showered when it was pointed out to me that I looked and smelled like a man in the grip of a severe depression. I have a photograph of me in those day. The eyes give me away. They are not the thousand-yard stare eyes of the Christopher Walken cliché.* Far from being emptied of feeling, they overflow with fear.

I read about the case of the Canadian general Roméo Dallaire, force commander of the UN's Assistance Mission in Rwanda during the genocide, who, on his return, descended into suicidal despair. He turned to alcohol. He self-harmed with a razor. At one point he found himself driving his car at 150km/h on a Quebec road, with young children in the back, hoping for an 'accidental' death. The general wrote two memoirs of his Rwandan experiences and their aftermath, including one that dealt specifically with the PTSD that he suffered and which led subsequently to his medical release from the army. The smell of death had entered 'the pores of my skin', he wrote.[2]

Again, I do not compare my experience of Rwanda to his. But I was also coping with the weight of all the other wars, from childhood in the sixties to the battlefields of the new millennium. The sky of those last days was darker than any I knew before. The trees were barer. I imagined their branches wrapping and strangling me. I became paranoid. I thought Rwanda, in some shape or form I could not imagine, would reach out from the past to destroy me.

I was referred by my GP to the psychiatrist who treated me when I was in rehab. Dr Niall Campbell was my honest Ulsterman, a Ballymena Presbyterian with a laconic humour, an

---

* Christopher Walken appeared as a heavily traumatised veteran in Michael Cimino's Vietnam War film *The Deerhunter* (1978). Walken's character was shown playing Russian roulette for money, replaying the traumatic experience he suffered as a prisoner of the Viet Cong.

acute and unsentimental intelligence, and boundless compassion. At our first appointment he ran through a PTSD checklist.

Had I experienced a life-threatening event? – Yes

Did I experience nightmares and/or flashbacks? – Both

Did I experience arousal symptoms, i.e.: jumping at noises, memories stirred by smells etc? – Both

Did I feel persistent anxiety? – Absolutely

Had my mood changed? ... – Yes

I'm sure there were more, but that is all I remember. 'I think we can say you pass the test,' he said.

It was Gordon Duncan, my old alcoholism counsellor and now close friend, who brought me to hospital. I entered the doors of the Priory and went through the same routine as I had years before during rehab, except this time they were not looking for drugs or booze I might use to get stoned, but for medication that might help a soul intent on self-harm.

This was a darker place of the mind. With alcohol 'all' I needed to do was stop drinking. Keep talking to other drunks, do my AA meetings, and there was a fair chance I would stay sober. It isn't as easy as that for many people. I know this. But compared to PTSD that path felt beautifully simple.

I watched the alcoholics in the canteen each day. I envied their camaraderie, the routine and purpose of their programme. To go out to the garden I needed to get permission and sign a register. There had been people who fled the building and took their own lives. I was not going to do that and my conditions were soon relaxed, but I spent my first two nights on a mandatory suicide watch in a room near the nurses' station, where new arrivals could be more easily monitored. Lying there I felt ashamed, worthless and exhausted. I was shown immense solidarity in those days. My hand was held in that deepest moment of despair. Out of respect for the privacy of others, I can only write anonymously, but the love I was shown remains an act of the greatest generosity.

In a few days I emerged from the hibernation of suicide watch. There were shy encounters at the breakfast table. So many conversations started with 'What are you in for?' I met people suffering from severe depression, bi-polar disorder, obsessive compulsive disorder; people who were running from misery on the outside; even a kid who was running from the cops, because of his family's criminal history. He figured a psychiatric hospital would give him a break from the pressure he was under to become a state witness. Another patient – a young woman who smiled constantly – had set up a shrine to her cats and placed food there every day. There was nothing unusual about this. Who could scorn another's idiosyncrasies in a place like this? Not me who visibly jumped every time a door slammed or ground my face into the ground when the big army Chinook helicopters flew over the hospital on their way across London.

At weekends families and friends came.

After writing this sentence I stop. I stop for several hours. *Families and friends.* How could I ever accept sympathy, when I know the cost of my chosen life on those closest to me, the fear that they did not deserve.

I wanted to be a better man. I was introduced to group therapy for those experiencing PTSD. I sat with soldiers, abuse victims, car crash survivors, murder witnesses, and mostly listened. My best friends were an oil company executive who had cracked under the pressure of work, and a squaddie who had fought in Afghanistan and whose angry outbursts were getting him into trouble.

The therapist in charge of the group was a Spaniard, the daughter of a Republican exile of the Spanish Civil War. Cristina Garcia-Llavona did not treat her patients as fragile victims. She was willing to challenge us, however gently, when we tried to isolate and avoid the issues which brought us to hospital. I was glad not to be treated as a victim. I have always operated by the maxim that the only therapist who is good for me is one who will challenge me. My defensive tactics of avoidance, obfuscation, and intellectualising did not work with Cristina. I also started to see her as my one-to-one therapist.

It was only after working together for the best part of a decade that I learned her childhood ambition was to have been a war correspondent. She believed it was a way of helping people. I am not sure the years of listening to my emotional struggles convinced her that any help given was a price worth paying.

Cristina took the best of therapies available and crafted her own style of working, based on the needs of each patient. We used CBT (cognitive behavioural therapy) where the work is, at its most essential, an attempt to replace negative thoughts with positive ones. We worked on Rwanda using EMDR (eye movement desensitisation and reprocessing) – a technique that involves rapid movement of the eyes as a means of processing trauma. It came about when the psychologist Francine Shapiro was walking through a park in 1987 and found that by moving her eyes she could reduce the impact of painful memories. The American psychiatrist Dr Bessel van der Kolk, a pioneer in the treatment of PTSD, has written enthusiastically of the effects of the treatment: 'EMDR loosens up something in the mind/brain that gives people rapid access to loosely associated memories and images from their past. This seems to help them put the traumatic experience into a larger context or perspective.'[3]

I was desperate to stop the anxiety and depression. I read up on the scientific debates and concluded that I was willing to try anything – short of alcohol or psychotropic drugs – that could alleviate the pain. Being an addict, I did not trust myself around potentially addictive substances. I managed to handle sedatives on the highly stressed occasions when I needed them, but I had no idea how I would respond if I found a drug that suddenly managed to take the pain away.

I suggested to my psychiatrist that I undertake electric shock treatment. I had convinced myself that electricity might – as it were – zap the pain. I had seen fellow patients return from ECT looking dazed and exhausted, but a few told me it had lifted them from the darkness of deep depression. But the doctor demurred. Stick to what I was doing with Cristina, he said. Trust the process.

So, I relied on EMDR. In practice it meant sitting with Cristina and recalling my Rwandan experiences while she tapped out her metronymic rhythm on my hands. I went back to the roads of 1994, back to the smells, the cadavers in the rivers, the remembrance of a road where we spotted – just in time to turn around – men preparing an ambush. It took me back to the faces of the living, the killers and the doomed, back to who I was then, in all my relentless energy and craziness. It ended, always, with a journey to my safe place. I cannot say EMDR cured me. But it took me safely into and out of places I would have unhealthily avoided for the rest of my life.

It was less easy to confront the sense of human failure I felt after Rwanda, the question of 'moral injury'.

I was convinced that my courage had failed me. The ambition to be heroic, which I had cherished as a child, ended in the town of Butare. I learned that many of the people we had filmed at the *Préfet*'s office in Butare were murdered in the fortnight after we left. One account describes how they were crowded onto buses, even forced into the luggage compartments, under the eyes of Préfet Nsabimana – the man whom I believed at the time represented a glimmer of decency – and then driven away to be killed. I met a Butare survivor in the Rwandan capital Kigali years later. She had been raped by the Interahamwe and was now suffering from AIDS. The woman remembered the white television crew coming and thinking that she might be about to be taken to safety.

It is reasonable to ask what possible intervention we might have made that could have saved the lives of the people outside the prefecture, or if even thinking we could have altered their fate was delusional.

I spoke about guilt with Cristina.

'Who do you think you were back then?' she asked. 'Did you truly believe you could have been the big saviour? Were you so powerful and important?'

With these words Cristina hit on a painful truth of my personality. Yes, there was a perfectly understandable feeling of sadness to discover what happened to the people at the prefecture. I am sure my colleague David Orr felt the same when he visited Tutsis imprisoned at a camp outside the town of Gitarama. But sorrow, even a lingering feeling of helplessness, is very different from the idea that I could have acted as a saviour, that there was some gesture – perhaps even of martyrdom – I could or should have undertaken that would have redeemed the terrible situation of those June days in 1994. One writer on the psychology of guilt puts it well: 'Guilt is defined, from a psychological perspective, as a "feeling of responsibility or remorse for some offence, crime, wrong, etc … whether real or imagined." The key part of that definition for me is the fact that guilt stems from this deep-seated belief, or desire, that we are much more powerful in a moment than we actually are. Often times it is the belief that we could've done something to prevent the situation, even though in reality we couldn't. It's grandiose.'[4]

If I was willing to believe that I could, somehow, have saved those people then I was back to the hero fantasies of my childhood. With Cristina's help I could see that there was nothing tangible we could have done, short of setting up camp with the refugees – without supplies of food and water – and hoping the militia would not kill us too. Even if we had had a satellite phone – we did not – who were we going to call? The United Nations, that had abandoned the people already? At the time I was so frightened that the thought of making a stand never occurred to me. I just wanted to get out of Butare.

There are all kinds of things you imagine doing when you are in a place of safety. But Rwanda was a place of maximum danger. It demanded that every sense was tuned to the potential for death. It was a place consumed by evil. I have long wrestled with the idea of 'evil' as a genuine presence rather than a hyperbolic adjective to describe those who do terrible things. But evil is not the opposite of good. Nor is it some metaphysical presence, destined to be sensed but not understood. Evil is an absence – of moral courage, kindness, humanity.

In the years after the genocide, I believed that the apocalypse that descended on Rwanda was something that could ultimately only be understood through recourse to philosophers and moral theologians. I looked to God for answers and to blame. This was mistaken. If I continued to see evil as something supernatural, a haunting if you like, if I believed there was an essential darkness in the human soul, I was giving up on hope and on my own recovery. Evil is not mysterious. What we call inhuman in the case of Rwanda – the recourse to mass murder of a perceived enemy, using methods calculated to terrorise – is intrinsically human. Brutal, cruel, pitiless, all of these yes, but completely within the bounds of what we know, and have always known, about human behaviour. Genocide is not the realisation of the unimaginable. Subject the human personality to a sequence of traumatising events and processes – in the case of Rwanda the collapse of prices for cash crops, the displacement of tens of thousands by civil war, the rise of hate media with its relentless demonisation of the minority as an existential threat, the ruthless determination of an ethnic elite to monopolise power, a colonial history of divide and rule, a long culture of obedience – and it becomes all too possible for the unimaginable to be imagined into being.

The Canadian writer and politician Michael Ignatieff, who visited Rwanda in the wake of the catastrophe, and with whom I later spoke, placed genocide in a context that helped to free me from metaphysical explanations about the human condition.

> This exterminatory impulse is much misunderstood. It is actually a kind of longing for utopia, a blood sacrifice in the worship of an idea of paradise. What could be more like paradise on earth than to live in a community without enemies? To create a world with no more borders or watch-posts, a world freed from fear in the night and war by day? A world safe from the deadly contaminations and temptations of the other tribe? What could be more beautiful than to live in a community with people who resemble each other in every particular? We all long for harmony, for an end to the seemingly interminable discord of human relations. What could be more seductive than to kill in order to put an end to all killings?[5]

For the sake of my mental health it was necessary to wrest Rwanda back into the realm of the factual, something I had attempted to do back when I interviewed the killers. Genocide was something to be understood, and potentially prevented by those with the capability to act. That it would almost certainly return, if not in Rwanda, then someplace else, was not my responsibility. I was not the United Nations Security Council. By following Cristina's advice on abandoning guilt, I could work to shorten the shadow which Rwanda had cast over my life.

After that, on the advice of my psychiatrist and therapist, I withdrew from reporting on Rwanda. If news from Rwanda appeared on my social media the old churn returned. I avoided anything to do with the place. I blocked emails containing the word Rwanda, likewise on social media. I was wary too of solipsism. A tragedy which had claimed the lives of up to 800,000 people and then sparked a vast conflict in central Africa claiming the lives of millions, was a story of Rwandan and Congolese suffering, not a narrative onto which to project the emotional trauma of one white man. I was suffering from PTSD before I ever got to Rwanda. It had certainly deepened my mental health problems, but it was not to *blame*.

I was shadowed by the memory of those who had witnessed the murder of their families, endured rape, and mutilation, and unlike me had no access to medication or therapy. I did not want to discuss the Rwandan experience, even with close family and friends. I avoided Rwanda to break an attachment that was destructive, but also because I was still afraid – as if Rwanda retained an otherworldly power that might yet reach out and finish me off.

Never mind that avoidance is a core symptom of PTSD, something Cristina gently reminded me of. As the US government

Veterans' Affairs Department puts it: 'If you go out of your way to avoid thoughts, feelings, and reminders related to a traumatic event, your symptoms may get worse.'[6] But after EMDR, and by giving Rwanda a wide berth, I did experience a real improvement in my symptoms for a while. They did not disappear, however. Nor did my longing for the wars.

I was doing less war reporting. I did not join the colleagues being smuggled into Syria. A risk too far. But I could have moved on from conflict reporting after 2008, perhaps found a job as a presenter on TV or radio. Yet whenever it was suggested to me, I reacted defensively: 'That's not me. I'm a reporter. I'd go fucking nuts in a studio.' Which might have been true, but my reaction spoke loudly of the hold that war still exercised.

It endured even after an incident in which a cameraman and dear friend, Tony Fallshaw, disappeared while working with me in Bangui, the capital of the Central African Republic, at the time a wilderness of warlords competing in viciousness. He had gone to pick up some general shots at a church which had been attacked a few days earlier by a Muslim militia. But for several hours there was no reply from his phone or that of our security advisor or the local producer. They failed to meet their appointed arrival time at the hotel. This was out of character. Tony and the security advisor, Rich Stacey, an ex-paratrooper, were dependable people with immense experience. We called Tony's number repeatedly until it was eventually answered by a laughing, and probably stoned, voice which declared that 'Tony is dead.' I pictured him lying on the streets of a slum. I felt sick. I knew from experience how possible it was. So possible. As easy as bad luck. My legs started to go from underneath me and I slumped on the bed. How would I tell their families? *Not another dead friend. Please God no, let this not be true.*

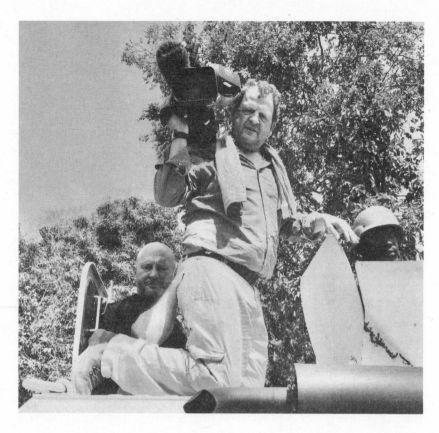

Comrades in all the wrong places: Richard Stacey and Tony Fallshaw.

It was in fact a hoax call by the militia. The team had been held by five gunmen. Grenades were produced. They were robbed and threatened with violence, but were eventually let go. I could only think I was lucky, they were lucky. Lucky now, but who says always?

Wars big and small were calling everywhere in those days. In the Middle East the Islamic State Caliphate rose out of the folly of the American war in Iraq and the decades of brutalising history under Saddam before that. Colleagues were being kidnapped and butchered on camera. War seemed more dangerous than ever before. The murderous hatred directed at journalists as a group was something I had not previously known. I reported from the Kurdish positions facing IS in Iraq, and saw the aftermath of a suicide bombing in Kirkuk. The killers were all around. I cannot remember the rationalisations I used to go to that front line. Maybe I had even given up offering excuses.

Then history shifted. War returned to Europe. A few hours flying time from London, the unfolding conflict in eastern Ukraine drew together my preoccupations – history, identity, trauma, and how they mark human lives. I went east.

15

East

Child of the fields
The wide fields
The flower fields
The fields of the sun
We found you
On a narrow road
Near Hrabove.

Child whose hair
Riffled
And stilled
In the July breeze
Whose broken shape
A passer-by
Had seen at dawn
And covered
With a pillowcase.

Child forsaken
Whose parents
Lay beyond
Where the fields
Burned still.
I placed sunflowers
At your feet
And prayed.

Child
Who returns to me now
Five years later
On a road in the Drôme
Where a late sun
Ignites the olive trees.

Oh Child
Forgive me
I wish
I could unsee you.

Written by author, 7 August 2014

In July 2014, twenty years since the end of the summer of slaughter in Rwanda, I was standing once again in an expanse of ground beside the bodies of the mutilated dead and asking if the evidence of my eyes could be believed.

These were the victims of a war initiated by President Vladimir Putin in the spring of that year, after Ukraine rejected the idea of living under the effective control of Russia. You could indulge all the arguments about it being caused by NATO expansion, but only if you wanted to obscure the central fact: an authoritarian bully, dreaming of a new Russian imperium, decided Ukraine had no right to exist as a state independent of Moscow's domination.

There were some unpleasant characters and military outfits on the Ukrainian side. One of my most uncomfortable encounters during the conflict was with the ultra-nationalist Pravyi Sektor (Right Sector) whose thugs held us at their checkpoint late one night outside Donetsk.* It was one of those moments when – for a few moments – anything might have happened. Beating, even shooting. But the persuasive powers of Daryna and Sasha got us through.

I had been working with Daryna Meyer since the first days of the war. She is from Donetsk but was forced to leave after threats from the rebels. They do not like the BBC and took it out on her. Leaving meant uprooting her mother, brother and sister, and her two-year-old-son. The ranks of Ukrainian producers are dominated by such women, conspicuous for their tenacity and physical courage. Daryna also brings kindness to her work. She is a loving person, and the victims of war appreciate this.

This time I was going because Ukraine had just become the biggest story in the world. Malaysian Airlines Flight MH17 had been shot down on 17 July 2014 at twenty minutes past four in the afternoon, killing 298 people, among them eighty children.

On that afternoon I was in Istanbul, tired and happy after hours of clear-water swimming on the Princes' Islands and slow

---

* Far-right groups, like the Azov Battalion and Pravyi Sektor, were among the most effective fighting units during the early stages of the war. Azov was eventually absorbed into the National Guard and began to draw its members from beyond the ultra-nationalist fringe. But the far-right was nothing like the defining force in Ukraine that Russia and its apologists like to pretend. They were scary and brutal on an individual level, but Ukraine is not run by fascists.

wandering by the shoreline. I was in the middle of lunch when the phone call came telling me of the disaster. I decided straight-away – without thought of what might lie ahead or what would have to be cancelled and who let down and who made afraid – that I would go as quickly as I could to eastern Ukraine. No matter that I was in a place of peace then and could have said no.

'We couldn't have stopped you,' Cristina said to me later. 'Nobody had any control over you. You would make excuses to go to the war. You were constantly bargaining. There was always a "right reason" to go to where it was dangerous. You were unstop-pable. You were like a toddler trying to put his hand in a fire.'[1]

The day after the plane crash I was travelling east, crossing the Dnipro, counting the smaller rivers and solitary figures fishing. The rain came in sweeping heavy downpours, flattening the sunflowers and corn. The dead civilians had been killed by a missile system that had been driven across the border from Russia and most likely operated by Russian personnel. Afterwards the lies and conspiracy theories flowed freely. I won't repeat them here. Giving expression to lies has become a form of complicity. The dead were the dead of Putin's war.

At the main rebel checkpoint before Donetsk a soldier asked what we thought would happen next. He seemed frightened. Would the Americans attack? I said I doubted it. He waved us through.

We came from the direction of Donetsk along back roads from which the usual rebel checkpoints had vanished. Had they gone because of shame over the disaster, or from fear of retribution? Whatever their motive, we felt relief. There would be none of the ritual harassment, ordering us from the vehicle for endless searches and scrutinising of passports with the threat of arrest and deten-tion in one of their numerous basement jails. At the back of our minds always was the experience of the *Sky News* team who were hauled off into the woods and subjected to a mock execution, or the observers from the OSCE – Organisation for Security and Co-operation in Europe – who ended up held hostage in a basement by the mayor of a small town.

There was no other movement on the roads. On the way to the crash site at Hrabove we passed field after field of sunflowers. 'When will they harvest?' I asked Sasha.

'Next month. They look nearly ready,' he replied.

Sasha, always even-tempered and always kind, with his broad, smiling, eager face, his children now in their early twenties and each in solid relationships of which he approved, and counting the days until he could go home to the wife he dearly loved and whom he called several times a day as we traversed the battle zones of eastern Ukraine. Before the war he had driven for tourists and business people and once, to his great pride, for the pop group Boney M. on their Ukrainian tour.

I had asked Sasha about the sunflowers because I did not want to think about what might lie ahead of us. Deflection, distraction, avoidance. Sensing this he began a monologue about how the crop is produced, the mechanisation of the life of the fields, how it had all changed since the time of his grandfather, who had known the collective farms and Stalin's famine, which killed millions and helped shape a Ukrainian identity that looked on Moscow as the citadel of tyranny.

Sasha stopped talking. There was a shape on the side of the road about a hundred yards ahead. It was lying amid the sunflowers, covered in a white sheet. There were smears of blood on the sheet. Somebody had covered the remains and placed sunflowers around the body and moved on, presumably hoping the ambulances would come and retrieve whatever lay underneath the covering. A tiny fringe of brown hair peeked out from underneath. As we drew closer we could see the body was that of a toddler, blown here by the force of the blast, in a place where we could see no other corpses. The child's parents had fallen to earth elsewhere, possibly at the main crash site that lay ahead of us, about a mile or so away, according to Sasha.

A vehicle approached from the direction we had come, an ambulance heading to the crash site. A ramshackle contraption, it stopped beside us, the engine running. The driver was exhausted as if he had driven through the night to reach this point, an out-of-towner from one of the other rebel cities, called in to help in the aftermath.

Sasha asked if he would take the toddler. 'We are here for the living,' the man replied, and drove on. There was nothing we could do for the dead child. Sasha was sure the local recovery teams would arrive later and take the body.

We left and went in the direction of the plateau at Hrabove where Flight MH17 had been shot down and where the bodies of the passengers lay scattered across a radius of twenty miles, some on ground blackened by the fire from the crash, others in wheat fields, their positions marked by staves of wood onto which pieces of white cloth had been tied.

Out of the car the air smelt of jet fuel and death. Twenty-four hours after the crash small fires were still burning. I saw the plane's cockpit section, where the pilots had been killed instantly by the blast from the Russian missile; the corpse of a man strapped into his seat, one hand raised in the air in the shape of a fist; the remains of a brown-haired woman, her body twisted in the still smouldering wreckage; lumps of fuselage. A woman's red hat, a set of playing cards, toys, a child's diary; more bodies and parts of bodies.

A journalist came down the road and said: 'No problem find-ing meat for dinner.' At the time I was speechless. Looking back, I am more understanding. I think they were in shock. The joke was a defence against the horror.

I made notes, as if the writing down of all that I could see would put the facts at a distance. I have always struggled not to think of what the victims of violence were feeling in those moments when death loomed. The report of the Dutch investi-gating team (Flight MH17 had flown from Amsterdam) revealed that the cockpit had fallen first. The rest of the plane continued to fly on for another five miles. It took approximately one and a half minutes from the moment of the explosion for the fuselage and the passengers to hit the ground. As the Dutch report put it: 'The impact was entirely unexpected, which means that people were barely able to comprehend the situation in which they found themselves.'[2]

Did the women, children and men who lay around me in the fields know that they were doomed, or were they taken by a violent spasm that obliterated consciousness? I hoped that it was sudden.

It took a year for the report to come out. I remember turning to the pages that dealt with the passengers' fate: 'There was hardly any time for a conscious response,' it said.

A number of occupants immediately sustained severe injuries as a result of the factors, probably causing death. For others the exposure caused reduced awareness or unconsciousness. It could not be ascertained at which moment the occupants died, but it is certain that the impact on the ground was not survivable.[3]

Human remains would be found in the fields for up to a week after the crash. A fat militiaman whom we nicknamed 'Grumpy' held sway over the site, pointing his automatic rifle at anyone who challenged his authority, or who even sought to move further up the road. Before the war he drove a lorry. I asked him if the horror all around us would persuade him to stop fighting. He dismissed my question: 'You're only here because foreigners are dead. Where were you when our kids were being killed?'

I had been present. In Donetsk and Mariupol and Odesa on the Black Sea, when those he called his people were dying. He paid no attention. Who cared where I was and for the outpourings of a fraught reporter at the scene of mass killing?

Later that day I lost my professional distance. A group of international ceasefire observers had arrived. There was no ceasefire to observe. Shelling and rocket strikes echoed in the distance. After a hold-up of several minutes while Grumpy gave them his grievance-filled lecture, the observers proceeded along the tar road, past the wreckage and past the dead, some of whom had been brought from the fields and placed in black body bags. Several were only partially covered. We passed a young man. He had fair hair and his face appeared unmarked, but all of his clothing had been stripped away by the force of the explosion or the power of the winds as the plane careened through the sky at over 500 miles an hour. There were militiamen, observers, journalists, all of us walking past in a group of perhaps thirty. I thought how obscene, our passing in silence this dead young man lying exposed.

I stopped a militiaman and pointed to the body. 'You cannot let him lie uncovered. Cover him please,' I pleaded.

There was a moment of connection. He looked towards the dead man and then called one of his men and gave orders for a body bag to be brought to the site. The young man was sealed from view, but I still see him as he was that morning – fair-haired, death pale and naked – before the plastic closed over his face. He was placed in an ambulance and driven to the railway station at Kharkiv, where he was loaded into a goods wagon with the hundreds of others and carried through the night to a mortuary where the dead would be identified and sent home, ten days after the jet crashed from the sky over the fields of Hrabove.

The women of the village brought flowers. They stood with the priest, portly Father Oleg, who led them in prayer, clustered around a stone cross and standing directly opposite where one of the plane's wheels and one of the engines had come to rest. Dust from the blackened ground blew in our direction. Some of the women were crying. One said she was afraid of what might follow the catastrophe: 'It does not feel safe here.' Father Oleg said the people were filled with anguish for the dead. He asked us to follow him to his little church, a short drive away through the cornfields. There he gave each of us a laminated photo of an icon of the Blessed Virgin and Infant Jesus and asked that we remember the villagers as people of peace. He picked plums from the small orchard opposite the church and apologised that these were the only hospitality he could offer.

We went back to the crash site over the next week. One day we took a wrong turn on our way back and drove into a valley where the Ukrainian air force was bombing rebel positions. The rebels fired in our direction, warning shots that skimmed over the roof of our car and forced us to stop. Men ran down to the road from a dugout. They screamed at us. We held our arms out the windows. *No threat. You see. No threat.* With this, they waved us on.

* * *

I am scared all the time now but do my best to keep it hidden. With each expedition it gets harder. But I keep going. I cannot stop myself. You are maybe asking yourself now, because I am, how was I carrying this when I got home? With difficulty, is the answer, with colossal amounts of mental absence, with Xanax and zolpidem to get through the night, with all the effort I could muster to be present and try to be the father I needed to be. There were periods of outward stability where I could do normal things, seem normal to others. I could cook good meals and laugh at dinner tables. But the gloom was always waiting its moment inside me. I would sense it rising and follow the instinct I knew and run to the wars.

There is a winter morning when we are close to rebel positions near Donetsk airport. Not a soul can be seen. The trees are freshly shredded by shrapnel. Impact craters cover the ground and pit the road. We come up against a mound of earth that blocks our way. For a few seconds we sit wondering what to do next. The Ukrainian incoming fire starts. Shells really do scream when they come over your head. I am thinking about this when Richard Stacey shouts at us to get into cover. I trust 'Stace' to take over when things are bad. This is very bad. We scramble out of the van. The rebels have dug trenches along the roadside. I run, stumble, and fall into a trench. I hear the cameraman, Tony Fallshaw, roar 'incoming' and another shell whistles over and detonates a short distance away. The ground vibrates. I press my head into the earth. The others seek their own cover. The gunners are clearly targeting us. They have found their range. I remember my training. *Eat the earth. Press your body into any hollow. Hope they fire nothing that explodes overhead.* Stace realises our Ukrainian producer, Daryna, has gone back to the van to fetch a colleague's press identification. He runs back to the vehicle and pulls her to a trench.

I pray fast. *Christ, let it just be random harassing fire. Let it not be a full-on pounding.*

The shelling stops after three or four rounds. In the pause, Stace calls out our names – call and response – to see if everyone is alive and where we are. He describes our predicament in a few words: 'We can stay here and wait for those fuckers to start up again, which they will, or we can make a run for it.' The trench is no guarantee of safety, and how long could we wait out here in the freezing cold? Night offers no sanctuary. The Ukrainian gunners can still easily pick up our movements after dark.

Again, that waiting, that nerve-ravaging listening for the sound of incoming. We run to the vehicle and Sasha races us back along the road towards the city, passing people outside a block of flats – those too old or too tired or too lacking in resources to move into the city and away from the front line.

As soon as we reach the hotel I go to my room. I lie on the bed, shaking. A knock at the door. Stace stands in the corridor.

'Are you doing okay, mate?'

I shake my head.

'Let's have a cup of tea.'

He comes in and we sit and drink tea. Stace was blown up in Northern Ireland and still carries the scars. On the surface of things we don't look as if we should have much in common. But war has a way of eliminating anything but what you really need to know about someone: if it all falls apart can I depend on them? I cannot remember now what we talked about. It didn't matter. The terror passed.

Although anxious about what might lie ahead, I have always loved the journey east: Kyiv station in the pre-dawn dark, snow falling, the trains filled with soldiers heading to the front; old people hauling their shopping after a weekend visiting their children in the capital. The fields that run forever into the whiteness of a land that rolls east as far as the Pacific, north to the Arctic Ocean, south to the Sea of Azov and the Black Sea, and how in spring they transform into golden grain and sunflowers alert to the radiance of the morning.

Anton Chekhov was beguiled by the beauty of the Ukrainian steppe. He wrote of how 'the grass drooped and life stood still. The brownish-green and sunbaked hills appearing lilac from afar …'[4] This was the pre-motorised world of the Russian imperium, before the fleets of combines rumbled across the collective farms and obliterated stillness; it was before Stalin starved millions and before Hitler's armies set the east on fire.

Now, two years after the loss of Flight MH17, the fields of the front-line zone are fallow. Nobody is left to bring in the harvest.

We pass the rusting wreckage of a tank. Somebody has placed a garland of fresh flowers where soldiers died. We are moving during a lull in the fighting. I listen to birds calling from the bushes that surround the entrance to a farm. The house has been abandoned. It is a broken-down miserable little affair. The front door is open, but I do not enter. There may be booby traps. In the gloom beyond I see several bags of rotting potatoes spilled on the floor, blankets, a shovel. The owners left in a hurry.

This close to the front, calm is the greatest enemy. It has often betrayed us. When the shelling stops the body's craving for normality takes over. You are still watchful but gradually the breaths become longer, the body untenses from its tangle of tight nerves. In the spring fields it is surprising how birdsong and the hum of insects quickly reasserts itself as the dominant noise. But then, when you have drunk some water and lit a cigarette, slumped against a wall, and started to talk in normal voices about anything that comes into your head, it starts again.

Loud cracks and flashes in the fields nearby, a surge of adrenaline and shouts of 'Go, go, go' in English and Ukrainian. The van door slams, and we are hurtling back the way we came. A mile down the road we stop next to a hotel. It is closed but we are able to park up in the empty lot at the front. Why do we think a mile will make any difference? The rebels have artillery that can travel thirty miles. We huddle and discuss. How close were the incoming rounds? Maybe 300 metres from the road? We figure they were aiming for the Ukrainian base and not the road. We were just unlucky to have stopped where we did.

There is a difficult choice. If we don't get to Piski today, we run out of time. The Ukrainians will not take us back down this road a second time. They have a war to fight, and we are a nuisance. The village of Piski is closed to the world. It has taken a lot of pleading and cajoling by Daryna to get us this far. I tell the team that nobody must feel pressured. If one person wants to leave, then we all leave. Nobody should feel ashamed, or that they are letting anybody down. The decision to keep going is unanimous, we have weighed up the odds. We turn our vehicles around and go back in the direction of the firing.

My mouth dries up. I stick my hands under my arms so that the others will not see them shake. But the energy is simply transferred to my shoulders. Do the others notice? I think, hope, that everybody is too preoccupied with watching and listening and the business of their own survival.

In the first months of war in early 2014, Piski swung back and forth between the two armies. The village mattered then because it was a rear base for the Ukrainians holed up in Donetsk airport and because it controlled the approach to the water supply at the

Karlivske reservoir. In July, after weeks of bitter fighting, a Ukrainian volunteer battalion has finally seized control. To the politicians and oligarchs who bankroll them, Piski is real estate in which enemies are to be pulverised. Their soldiers stalk each other through abandoned houses. They plant landmines and fire mortars and race to the bunkers when the other side fires back. Piski is the festering heart, the point where all the corruption, cynicism, courage and pointless death converge.

The war around Donetsk airport, of which Piski is a central part, has mutated into a series of local grudges: the people in the ruined village against those hiding in the factory; the sniper lying on the slag heap versus the mortar team trying to walk their bombs onto his position; the fighters in the trenches firing bursts at the people bringing in food; commanders screaming abuse and threats at each other on their radios. Headline writers are fond of calling this a forgotten war.

Not forgotten by those being made homeless and traumatised, or those who are doing the killing. Named after the composer Sergei Prokofiev, a native of the region, the international airport at Donetsk is a source of pride for Ukrainians. It was built to welcome football fans during the 2012 Euros but is now the epicentre of the war's madness. In the winter of 2015, the Ukrainian defenders are finally forced to withdraw after a five-month long siege, but traces of their dead lie around the ruined terminal. The remains of a soldier mulch into the earth near the main road into the complex. The essence of him has seeped away a long time ago. He is flattened out, just scraps of parchment skin that show through the ragged cloth of the uniform. But his boots are still intact, made of good leather that has endured the snows. A fragment of bone, yellowy white, sticks out awkwardly over the top of the right boot. The pro-Russian commander 'Givi' cannot say how long the body has been there. Nobody knows where the head has gone. It could have been blown to pieces or been carried off by animals. There are bits of people all over the airport. A few days before, Givi's thugs had forced Ukrainian prisoners to collect bodies and bits of bodies. They'd missed this one.

'You've got to get it cleared away,' he says to one of his own men. 'For fuck's sake, it's been here for weeks.'

Givi is the rebel who swore to liberate his land from the clutches of the 'fascist Ukrainian junta'. He is the psychopath who beats and humiliates prisoners, who cuts the insignia from uniforms and forces them into the mouths of terrified men in front of pro-Russian television cameras, the murderer who shoots people out of hand, and the martinet who gets angry when a corpse is left to rot too long. This has nothing to do with concern for the dignity of the dead. In the middle of that blasted landscape – with its shredded trees, shell holes, its bomb-wrecked terminal, where soldiers are fighting and dying still – that one body has upset his personal idea of order. Unusually squeamish, I think to myself, for a man with so much blood on his hands.

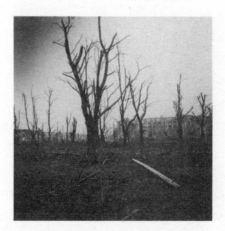

Donetsk airport in the winter of 2015.

Givi is about six feet tall, handsome, sinewy, with a slim mous-
tache. Think of a guitar-strumming balladeer in an amateur talent
show, or a ballroom dancer. It is customary in accounts of psycho-
pathic warriors to include a description of hollowed-out eyes – empty,
pitiless, cold. But Givi has the eyes of a lover. They implore,
seduce and cajole, and when he is angry, they flash with mad electricity. There is a murderous honesty about him that marks him
out among the shifting band of ideologues, criminals, chancers
and lunatics who have taken power in eastern Ukraine. If Givi
promises to kill you, he will try his best. If he says he will protect
you from attack by drunken or renegade rebels he will, similarly,
be as good as his word. This is my assessment.

Before the war Givi worked in a rope factory in the industrial
town of Ilovaisk, around forty kilometres from Donetsk, and
before that he served in the Ukrainian army, the same army whose
soldiers he now abuses. His parents are Georgian. So, the picture
emerges of this boy from somewhere else, a foreigner in the
Donbas, who also says that he has a speech impediment (though
this is not clear to me listening to him) – the outsider who now
has a chance to prove he belongs as much as anyone else. These

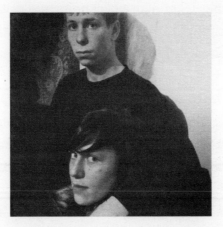

Faces in a Donetsk bomb shelter.

days I am highly attuned to the psychological state of the fighters I meet. But Givi, as far as I can detect, does not have PTSD. He acts out his variety of mental illness through imposing suffering on others. I do not want to cross this man.

It is no surprise to his soldiers or his enemies when he is killed in February 2017. Nobody is sure whether the job was done by a Ukrainian hit team, by Putin's operatives, or by an enemy in the rebel forces. Everyone I spoke to thought that Givi was living on borrowed time. The real 'crazies' like him can have a limited shelf life. Even the regime of venal goons who run Donetsk eventually became fearful of a man like Givi. His successor, another man of murderous habits, is also assassinated, it is rumoured by the Russians who weary of his ill-disciplined ways. On the rebel side of the lines there are echoes of the *Lord of the Flies* world I have come across in some of the African wars. I notice that I take more care around such people than I have done in the past. I would not now think of confronting them with the vehemence I displayed towards Rwandan war criminals. I am more fearful, no doubt of that.

We leave the big Ukrainian checkpoint under the Pervomaisk bridge. It has survived several direct hits from artillery. The men here are exhausted and wave us through with the warning: 'Go fast.'

Craters begin to appear in the road. Sasha swerves around them. There are clusters of shrapnel which can shred tyres in an instant. After five, ten, twenty minutes – my sense of time has vanished – we see an armoured personnel carrier parked across the road behind a barricade of concrete and sandbags. The Ukrainians are dug in around a villa. The roof and upper floor have been gutted by a direct hit. Downstairs, soldiers are crowded around a

stove, drinking tea. A teenager is clipping bullets into the magazine of his rifle. Above him is a sheet covered with the palm-prints
of schoolchildren in the Ukrainian colours, a patriotic gift offered
up by a headteacher. I climb a ladder into the burned-out section
of the building. From here the rebel lines are easily visible. Two
grain elevators about 300 hundred metres away make perfect
sniper posts.

Our military minder, Captain Yuri, is red-haired with a thick
beard, a girth that speaks of many good dinners, and the flushed
complexion of a man who lives a life that he loves. Back home he
has two young daughters who are the joy of his existence. 'And
my wife, I love her too!' he laughs.

He knocks his fist gently on my helmet. 'Keep this on. All the
time. And don't stand around in the open.'

A soldier wearing a keffiyeh wanders over. He is an experienced
fighter, a man in his forties with a watchful expression, alert to
every element of his surroundings. He will take us from the
command post to the forward trenches. Igor Phillipov was a landscape gardener before the war began. The others call him 'The
Spaniard' because of his dark looks. He volunteered when war
broke out. Igor knew Donetsk and Piski from his days as a driver
on the rally car circuit, a time he cannot easily imagine now.

I follow Igor through a warren of abandoned houses. 'Keep to
my exact line,' he says. Spent shell-casings glisten in the morning
sun. Sporadically the rifles open up, back and forth. A few
minutes' release of tension. Then the birds sing again as if nothing
has happened. Do birds get accustomed to war, I wonder. Can
they be traumatised? We lean against a wall. Some men are sitting
in a trench opposite ready to return fire if the noise starts up
again. They wave across to us, beckoning us to join.

I look at Stace for his guidance.

He says to wait. The closest rebels are only fifty metres away in their trenches. He is waiting to hear if a sniper fires. Igor starts to tell me his nerves are at breaking point: he needs to go home. He takes out two photographs. In the first he poses with his wife. She is blonde, petite and her arms are wrapped around his waist, her head leaning into his chest. They are on holiday, standing outside a restaurant in a cobbled street. The photograph has been taken by one of his sons. The two boys are in the next one, a tall lad who looks strikingly like his father, and the younger one with fairer hair who is closer in looks to his mother. 'A few days at home with them will fix me,' he says, hopefully. But he does not believe this. Home is far away. It gets further every day he spends on the line.

Our red-haired minder returns. He wants us to leave now, afraid the lull will soon end. 'I don't want you dead on my conscience,' he says. He laughs again, a deep-throated genuine laugh intended to give us confidence for the drive out. We obey his orders and race back down the road. A day later Captain Yuri, father of two daughters, is killed by a landmine.

I had only spent a day with him, but Yuri was a kind man, and now he is dismembered, in a body bag travelling back to his home town and a heartbroken family. I have not hardened, not a bit.

According to Susan Sontag, someone 'who is perennially surprised that depravity exists, who continues to feel disillusioned (even incredulous) when confronted with evidence of what humans are capable of inflicting in the way of gruesome, hands-on cruelties upon other humans, has not reached moral or psychological adulthood'.[5] But what of the obverse? The individual who is so immersed in that depravity that their vision of the world is warped, the person who sees only bad outcomes.

As the years have progressed it is that weight, as much as trauma itself, that has borne down on me with increasing force, and sent me to find in war the people who offer a contrary human narrative to that of Givi in Donetsk or the killers in Rwanda. I seek the friendship of kind people stranded in the zones of cruelty. The same goes for the people with whom I choose to work. It is their decencies I set against the accumulating poison of the wars, the moral injury that is as great a burden as my twitching face or sleepless nights. They become my antidotes, my spiritual support system, on the battlefields I cannot leave behind.

16

Trip Wires

Set the broken psalmic rhythm of rain
beneath your heart …
… Eastern Ukraine, the end of the second millennium.
The world is brimming with music and fire.

'So I'll Talk About It', Serhiy Zhadan[1]

Walking back into Piski we are with a soldier from a new rotation. He is young, a conscript, swearing away in his helmet and body armour and camouflage fatigues. He hates the place. 'I want to leave and go home.'

I think: *If anything happens this poor fucker is no use to us. He'll be gone.*

Halfway up a lane I lurch to a halt. A slender copper wire glistens on the ground. My heart accelerates. 'Trip wire!' I shout. Everybody freezes.

The soldier comes forward. 'Finished,' he says, 'old.' In fact, it is wire from a guided anti-tank missile. We step over and keep walking. My heart rate slowly recovers. There is firing up the road, about seven hundred yards away. The explosions are further off, around the airport.

There are just eighteen people left in Piski from a pre-war population of 3,000. The remaining residents are marooned inside concentric circles of devastation. Nobody moves in or out anymore. The place is ghost-ridden. At any moment a shell can land on your house. Why would anybody stay?

In trying to answer that question I come across a remarkable couple. Daryna meets them in Piski a week before I arrive. Up and down the empty streets she goes with Sasha, knocking on doors and calling out to see if anybody is home. Our plan is to make a short film on the last residents of this once thriving place. The first people who answer are Anatoly and Svetlana Kosse. All around them are the ruins of houses struck by shellfire. The steel door to their garden is punctured by bullets and shrapnel. But inside, apart from a blown-out window, there is order and brightness. 'Flowers, such flowers,' Daryna tells me.

Anatoly and Svetlana are both sixty-nine. They are fit and keep active with work around the house and on their vegetable patch. When we reach them a week later Anatoly is with his bees in the shade of some Linden trees at the back of the house. Svetlana is chopping onions. A feast is being prepared in our honour. They are people who have fun in their eyes. It is there when the afternoon light catches their faces. It picks out the laughter lines too. Anatoly looks as if he is perpetually on the edge of inviting you into an uproarious private joke.

The war is going on around us, but I feel safe. There is no logic to this feeling, but I accept it as a temporary grace.

'The honey is of good quality. We still have many bushes of flowers around here,' Anatoly tells me. In fact, since everybody left Piski the vegetation has grown abundantly. The gardens are left untended. There are no municipal workers anymore. Around his patch of vegetables (cabbage, potatoes, beans) are the craters caused by mortar fire. But nothing has touched his garden. 'It is just luck,' he says.

That night we have dinner by the light of candles. There is omelette, mashed potato, pickled cabbage, gherkins, home-made bread, juice from their own garden fruit. They tell me about their daughter who lives on the other side of the line in Donetsk. They worry about her. She worries about them. 'It is terrifying,' says Svetlana. 'Before, I only had a few grey hairs here.' She points to her head. 'And now you can see. When I look at myself with my glasses on, it is terrifying.'[2]

So why did they stay? Why did they not leave for the city?

At first Anatoly speaks of the bees. 'I am taking care of them, they are here, how can I just leave them?'

The working hive symbolises the civilised existence that they have struggled to maintain here. In this small patch there will be

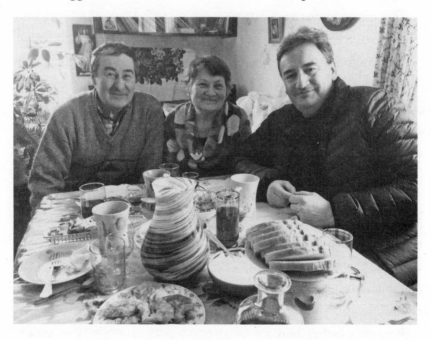

Anatoly and Svetlana Kosse with the author in Piski.

life. It will spring from the ground. It will sleep in winter and multiply in summer. The bees leave their hives to gather pollen from the overgrown gardens abandoned by the neighbours. Wild berries and settled plants tangle around each other. The weeds have grown high and press through the barbed wire placed at different intersections during the winter fighting.

Svetlana says she did evacuate to the city for several months, but Anatoly would not come. He feared the house would be looted. The couple pined for each other. 'When he was alone here, every morning and evening we called each other. I had a strong pain in my soul and so did he. He was a lonely man here because all the neighbours moved away.'

I ask Anatoly what his wife means to him. 'How can I explain what she means to me?' he says. Then he smiles and leans across and places his head on her shoulder.

The night is warm. We move outside and continue talking. There is outgoing mortar fire from the Ukrainians at the bridge. Tracer bullets speed across the sky like malign shooting stars. There are satellites winking far above. But there are no planes; nobody flies across here anymore. A bright light appears close to the Ukrainian lines. It is an unmanned drone, searching for targets. The gunners fire and try to bring it down before it can direct artillery fire.

They talk about happier days. Piski was where Svetlana grew up: a no-account, unspectacular village in the Soviet empire, where nothing changed, where terror and starvation existed only in the memory of her parents and grandparents. How could anyone back in the time of Brezhnev have pictured this chaos?

Anatoly's father had survived the Hitler war but died when Anatoly was just five years old, killed in an accident at the factory where he worked. That was in 1952, the year of Stalin's 'Doctor's Plot'* and of the birth of Vladimir Vladimirovich Putin.

They show us to our sleeping places and say goodnight. I decide to stay outside. I fear being buried in the rubble of the building if a shell comes in. It is idiotic. The same shell will still blow me to pieces outside.

It is cooler here. The young conscript sits on a chair smoking. I wake in the night and see that he is standing up, alert to the noise of vehicles. It is a heavy grinding sound. 'Tanks,' he says. They are up on the highway. It is impossible to know where they are going.

The following morning Svetlana brings me to see their neighbour, Sonya Tolmachova. 'She has a cow,' Svetlana says, 'and not much else.'

Sonya is slashing grass for winter fodder in the plot of land next to the beehive. When she has finished, she places it in a bag and drags it behind her. Sonya is seventy-eight and has a spinal deformity. She is bent almost double as she walks. Her own house, on the west side of Piski, closer to the front line, was destroyed in the opening weeks of the war. Since then, she has moved four times. This latest abode consists of a single small room in which she and her fifty-six-year-old son, Vladimir, live with several dogs. I cannot make out how many animals share the space; they come and go in a blur of barking and skittering paws. Vladimir has been severely disabled since shortly after birth: a doctor's mistake cut off the supply of oxygen to his brain for brief but essential moments.

---

* A group of Jewish doctors was falsely accused of planning to assassinate Stalin and other leading Soviet figures. Thirty-seven doctors were arrested and most subjected to torture. It is believed Stalin planned to deport the entire Jewish population of the Soviet Union to the Gulag in the wake of the plot. His death in 1953 brought an immediate end to the persecutions.

Vladimir's eyes are wide with panic when we enter the room. Sonya strokes his head and says softly: 'Don't be frightened, my little one. Nobody will take you away from me.' Our presence unsettles him. After a few minutes he calms. He lies on the bed gazing at the ceiling, from time to time pressing his fingers into the electric socket. He is safe from the danger of shock, as there is no power. Neither is there any hot water. A gas stove and heater provide the necessities of survival. When he is not poking the socket, he picks at his fingernails.

Sonya Tolmachova has one other child, a son younger than Vladimir, who was wounded at the start of the war and taken to hospital. She has no idea where he is now. Sonya says the soldiers bring food sometimes, and Anatoly and Svetlana call every day and bring vegetables.

They are waiting for us outside on the lane. Svetlana wants to give us some food for the journey. I thank them. I tell them that they help me. Through them I see another world that still contains kindness. Anatoly shrugs off the compliment: 'You make too much of us.'

As we drive away, they stand in the empty lane, waving and smiling.

I return in winter. Snow drifts rise on either side of the track. We have been moving east since dawn. The bridges are blown. The roads are bisected by trenches. The land is braided with tank traps and mines. But the railway keeps running. The war is two years old. It is hunched in the trenches that divide the land between the Dnieper and the Sea of Azov. It squats in basements and crumbling apartment blocks and stamps its feet in food ration lines on icebound mornings.

Last week at the Maryinka checkpoint a woman needed to go to the toilet. The queues to cross the line had reached five or more kilometres long. There were no facilities. She wandered a few yards into a field and vanished in flame and dust. A week later a minivan tried to jump the queue by heading into a field alongside the road. Four dead. The landmines have killed more than forty children. One hundred and nine others have been maimed.

How bland the facts. Calculate the legs, arms, all the body parts ripped apart in those explosions, and the minds forever wounded. Nobody advances, nobody retreats. The armies sit in their trenches and shoot without moving. They say the ceasefire holds.

The wind blows snow from the drifts into our faces. This is Akhmatova's wind 'gusting from the age of stone',[3] carrying with it the mutter of guns from the ruined factory at the top of the lane. The fighting is about seven hundred metres away. It will go on intermittently, a series of reflexive gestures from cold and bored men.

In the courtyard, standing with a few other people, I see a familiar face. Igor Phillipov 'The Spaniard' walks over. *By God*, I think, *he looks so much older*. We embrace. When I ask him what has changed, he replies: 'Now I just want to kill them all.'

There is no laughter. The landscape gardener who dreamed only of getting home to his wife and children is lost in a private war. He will not, or cannot, hold my gaze. I don't get the chance to ask what changed, what he saw or who he lost. He quickly says goodbye and jumps into a car with three other soldiers. They disappear towards the front. The few days at home did not cure his nerves. They never do. You just carry the sadness with you and plant it in someone else's garden. PTSD. Igor cannot leave the war behind. The only reality is this place, and the men around him.

*   *   *

I fly back to London after this trip. I spend time with my kids.

I am going to the wars less, but I cannot shake the agitation, an inner bristling, every time I watch colleagues reporting from war zones. After a few weeks the restlessness always starts again.

I keep going with the rationalisations.

But, what if...

We only spend an hour in the centre of Mogadishu?

We have really good armed security with us?

What if we only spend fifteen minutes at the front line in Donetsk?

What if there has been no shelling in the last two weeks?

What if the UN guarantees our security?

I repeatedly propelled myself back into danger with this kind of bullshit.

I was addicted, for all the reasons I've already laid out. I wanted to stop but I could not. I was like James breaking away when me and my artist friend tried to get him to stay in rehab. Not that I'd have admitted this to anyone. I came close a few times with Cristina, as far as saying there was 'an element of addiction'. Quite apart from the psychological stresses, I had become part of a stereotype: flak jacketed, helmeted, ducking to the sound of explosions, the wobbly camera shots as we ran, the story vanishing beneath the reporter's breathlessness. There was more to the world. There was more to me, I hoped. Partly to escape this trope, partly to try and avoid war. In 2017 I turned to a changing Africa.

17

Breakdown

Nobody can go back.
To go back is impossible in existence.

'Fear', Khalil Gibran[1]

Sudan was the first African country I ever visited. My earliest memory of it is of kindness. Nothing that happened in Darfur, or later in Khartoum, can erase that.

We were camping by the side of the road in the darkness, unable to travel further because the military checkpoint insisted that we wait for a senior officer to check our paperwork. That could not happen until morning. The desert was lit by starlight and the fires of truck drivers crossing the country between the Red Sea coast and Khartoum.

A man approached and extended a hand in greeting. From the other hand he offered a glass of tea. Still now I remember my first taste of that sweet, cinnamon-infused brew, and then the summons to join him and his friends by the fire. We had no mutual language and my driver's command of English was limited to basic phrases. We resorted to song. The crowd grew as other drivers drifted in from their fires to join us. I offered some Irish ballads, only marginally mournful. My host sang a song of a desert flower, the melody of which lives with me, though the words now are gone. It was the song of long-distance drivers, dreaming of their homes and loves, as they traversed the nearly 800-kilometre route between the coast and the capital on the banks of the Nile.

That night was long and largely sleepless: the desert ground was unyielding; feral dogs barked remorselessly in the shadows. But I did not feel unsafe. The truckers had taken me into their community. It was an African scene far more representative of the continent than the horrors I would subsequently spend so many years reporting.

A quarter of a century has passed since that encounter. Sudan has changed dramatically. Now, in the late spring of 2019, vast pro-democracy demonstrations have overthrown the dictatorship of President Omar al-Bashir. Tens of thousands of people are camped outside military headquarters in Khartoum. The scene is joyous. Ethnic differences are cast aside as people demand an end to autocracy. Nobody in the days of the dictator Colonel Nimeiri would have predicted the mass movement for democracy, not in the moribund years of Cold War autocracies.

Sudan is an example of a much wider shift. Across Africa, a vibrant civil society is emerging. There are websites, small newspapers, independent campaign groups on human rights, on climate, gender, and there are genuine elections in places that have only ever known dictatorships or stitch-ups. This is what drew me to apply for the position of Africa Editor at the BBC. Here was the chance to put the days of war behind me, to report on a different kind of history in the making. I also made it clear at the interview that I could not cover Rwanda. That would have to be done by somebody else.

I report on elections in Kenya and Congo, the release of political prisoners in Ethiopia, the overthrow of Robert Mugabe in
Zimbabwe, campaigns for the repatriation of cultural artefacts
looted by colonial forces in West Africa. There are old friends and
contacts to catch up with. I have the chance to mentor young
African journalists and learn from them. It feels like a liberation.
I am still travelling but not in fear.

It is all working, working well, until events intervene.

I am in Khartoum and it is only days since the massacre. Dozens
have been killed and raped by the militia. These are the same
people I had walked among a few weeks before – the chanting,
dancing, hopeful crowds with their music blaring from giant
speakers; the people who had come from as close as Omdurman
and as far away as Darfur, Blue Nile and Kordofan; university
students, market traders, civil servants, rugged farmers; the jazz
band weaving through the crowds at night on Martyrs' Square;
and all the others who came to look in wonder at the tented city
that encircled the Ministry of Defence and who told themselves
that in numbers there was strength. I did not see the horror that
was to come. Only once, leaving the demonstrations at the end of
the afternoon, did I have the sense that there was an alternative
possibility to the happy expectation of a peaceful transition to
democracy.

We pass through the security cordon erected by the demonstrators to keep out agents provocateurs. At the other end of the street
the militia lounge in their jeeps; as we pass there is laughter. I look
into the eyes of the gunman nearest to me and say: 'Salaam
Alaikum.' He does not respond but a comrade raises his hand
and, forming the shape of a gun, points in my direction. There is
more laughter. I keep walking.

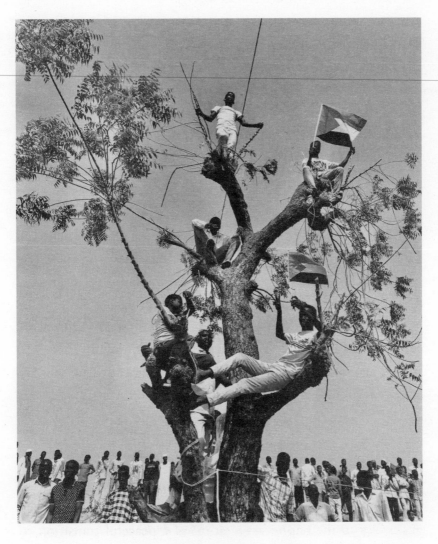

Days of Hope, Khartoum 2019.

On the night of 3 June 2019, the militia attack. I am back in London and am woken by a call from a friend in Khartoum. 'It has started,' he says, 'they are killing.'

I arrive a day later to a cityscape made silent by killing; where the jeeps of the militia, festooned with rocket-launchers, dominate every intersection and prowl the dusty back lanes. There has been mass shooting and bloodshed. Tents have been set on fire. The city of the people's revolution has been destroyed. Those who have escaped are in hiding across Khartoum and Omdurman.

I am given the address of a safe house in Omdurman where I am told I'll find survivors. We cross the Nile, weaving through the checkpoints of the militia. They are sprawling by the roadside in the heat, indifferent to our comings and goings. For they have nothing to fear from us; they are the undisputed victors. Their enemies are either dead or in hiding.

I am mindful of the dangers even so. I worry that the secret police might be following us, so they can discover who we are visiting. I imagine a scenario where they burst into the building and sweep up everybody present. We will be roughed up a little and then deported, brief 'heroes' of the free press, bemoaning the lot of 'our Sudanese friends' left behind, noble in our expressions of responsibility. But those taken with us will vanish into the torture chambers of the regime. It has echoes of Myanmar. There are security offices in the city with deep basements where people can scream for hours without being heard. Then there are the 'ghost houses', suburban homes turned into centres for the degra- dation of human beings. Here the animal cries can be heard by neighbours but, honestly, who is going to intervene against a regime like this? *Just turn on some music and pray for morning.*

I have already had a run-in with the militia. The day before we'd been taken on a government tour intended to show us build- ings looted by protestors. Our first stop – which turned out to be our last – was a clinic close by the river. There were broken windows, scattered files, X-ray machines smashed. The caretaker told us it was in fact the militia who'd done the destroying. Suddenly they arrived in the courtyard, crowding the journalists, haranguing the government minder. I felt my anger rising. 'Film them!' I urged the cameraman. My usually equable friend, Tony Fallshaw, raised his camera and grabbed a few seconds of footage. This only made the situation worse. Tony whispered in my ear: 'Not a fucking good idea, mate.'

The militia commander began screaming at us. Some of the other reporters were getting agitated with me. 'What the fuck, man?' said one. 'You'll get the whole lot of us locked up.' He was right and, knowing the militia, that would be one of the better outcomes. The minder spoke quietly to the commander. Gradually the tension subsided.

But I had shocked myself. I did not need a doctor to tell me that one of the defining symptoms of PTSD – a blinding rage – was at play here.

On the rutted streets of night-time Omdurman, I remain hyper-vigilant, constantly watching, looking out of the car's rear window. Only after we have navigated a series of lanes that take us deep into the suburbs do I begin to breathe more deeply.

The room is tiny. It smells of wounds going bad and the dried sweat of many people. I count twenty men in a space meant for no more than five. All have, so far, escaped the clutches of the regime. There are two empty beds just inside the door. I am bid to sit on one and offered tea. At the other end of the narrow room is another bed from which a man, wounded in the arm and leg, is staring at me. His eyes do not move. After a few minutes I understand that he is in a state of shock.

Another man ushers forward from the back of the group. He is introduced as an ambulance driver who has been ferrying the wounded to hospital during the massacre. I ask him to tell his story. He sits on the bed opposite me. He is so close that our knees touch.

I am from here, from Omdurman, and on the morning of the killings I went to help. I used my ambulance to take people to the hospital. But they would stop me sometimes and order out people and beat them. Sometimes they allowed them to get back into the ambulance after beating and at other times they did not. In the middle of the morning, I was going back to fetch more wounded people when I saw a young man carrying a woman who looked to be injured. They were stopped by group of militia. Maybe there was three or four of them. They started raping her. I drove with my ambulance to where it was happening, a short distance only. The militia went away when the ambulance came. When I got out, I saw that the woman they were raping was actually dead.[2]

I feel his body start to shake. A Sudanese colleague who's been translating the driver's story places an arm around him. At this gesture of tenderness the driver collapses, physically and loudly. He cries out and thrashes free of the translator's embrace, twisting and turning on the bed. We try to calm him, but he becomes more agitated. We hold his arms and legs, fearing he will harm himself and that his cries will bring the secret police to this hiding place. It looks as if he is having a seizure.

I run to fetch our security advisor, an ex-soldier with the British Army, who is outside watching the street for any sign of militia. A qualified field medic, he immediately takes charge tilting the head so that the man can breathe properly. His body's writhing begins to subside. When we leave, the driver is slumped against the wall, crying.

The best I can do is to ring a psychologist I know from a human rights organisation. She promises to send a volunteer to help the man if he wishes. But when our translator calls him the following morning, he declines the offer. He is back driving his ambulance. I have ignited great distress in this man by interviewing him. I have not manufactured the horrors in his head, but I have summoned them into a public space. Having done so I left him and returned home, as I've left so many others.

Alexander Dumas wrote: 'Moral wounds have this peculiarity – they may be hidden, but they never close; always painful, always ready to bleed when touched, they remain fresh and open in the heart.'[3] Khartoum reopened the wounds.

The breakdown comes one week after I return from Sudan, during a suffocating heatwave in France. They call it the *canicule* – the dog days – and it has been here for a week with no sign of lifting. We drive onwards along the Rhône and north through the Vendée, until we reach the vineyards of Alsace on the night of 24 July, the hottest night in France since records began. There are stops in small towns, service stations and country lanes so that I can get out of the car and try to control a rising panic. I ring my therapist but am unable to speak. Breathe in deeply, I am told, hold the breath for a few seconds and then slowly release. But the anguish does not abate. The tears come, unbidden and unending. I am constantly jumpy and snapping. I imagine being abandoned by all who love me. I turn to Xanax. One. Two. Three. This is the worst yet.

I lie awake all night in a small, rented house. My mind goes back and forth, an endless cycle of rumination. I know that if I pursue it long enough, it will lead to collapse.

What use am I?

You're nothing but a piece of shit. A burden. You're a fucking fraud. You're useless …

See all your wrongs … Go on, make a long list. Look at what you've done and what you've failed to do.

Live and suffer and pray that you are granted an early death …

I am to attend a wedding in the village of Thanvillé. It is a pretty place with woods all around and a lake in which to swim. There is a strange incident. I am sitting having coffee one morning when I hear shouting next door. It is a man's voice. The day before I saw a small child at the upstairs window. She did not look scared. It was more of a vacant look as if she was not really looking at anything. The man's shouting goes on and on. There is no response. I am roused from my Xanax torpor, concerned enough to go into the street and stand outside his house. It is louder there. I knock on the door and a short man in his thirties, tough-looking, comes out, and immediately takes the offensive.

'What's your problem?'

'No problem, I just heard shouting and wondered if everything was okay.'

'Everything is okay.'

'Are you sure? I heard very aggressive shouting and I am worried about the child.'

'I am shouting at a dog.'

'I see. If you are shouting at the child I would have to call social services. And shouting at the dog isn't such a good idea. You scare the kid and the dog.'

He is weighing up the situation. I suspect his instinct is to tell me to go to hell and slam the door in my face. But he is cunning. A call to the police would not be good for him. So he smiles. He tells me that it's the heat that has made him lose his temper. *Goodbye, mister. It will be quiet from now on.* And then he goes inside. I look up and the child is there again. There is no sign that she has been crying. There is nothing at all to see in her expression.

My rage is gone. I am now in a stage I know from the past. Fear and grief have blocked out all other feelings. From here it is a tranquilised fog. Without sedative medication I feel I will die from panic. I am hearing people like they are miles away.

I think: *You should be in hospital. It is not safe out here.* But I do not want to go back to hospital. *What would happen to me then? I'll end up destitute.* And so the rumination escalates until I see myself on the streets lying under cardboard, or locked away in a state psychiatric hospital guzzling medication to make sure nothing touches me anymore.

On the morning of the wedding, I swallow the requisite quantity of tablets, enough to guarantee that I won't disintegrate in front of everyone, but not so much that I appear utterly stoned. Everything happening now is happening inside my head.

In the garden of the Château de Thanvillé I smile and shake hands with people I do not know. I sit where I'm supposed to sit. Later I even dance, a kind of zombie shuffle.

I slip away from the wedding party when no one is looking and find a narrow road that leads into the hills above the village. It has rained in the afternoon. The immense heat has lifted. After about half a mile of walking, I spot a cemetery with row after row of black crosses: the graves of 607 German soldiers who died here during the Great War.

No one can disturb me here. For the first time in days, the pressure eases. I slump against the wall of the graveyard and fall asleep. I wake up after about an hour. I am driven home, silent, through the woods.

The following morning, I take a train for Paris at the station of Colmar. After a few minutes I hear an announcement telling me I am in fact on my way in the opposite direction, bound for

Switzerland. This is how it always starts. The unravelling of the basic details. Like it began on the trip to South Africa twenty-eight years ago, losing my money and tickets. Fixed facts begin to slip. The mind refuses to cooperate with plans.

I have only vague memories of what follows. A kind railway guard who helps me off the train and puts me on another bound for Paris. Dr Campbell in London with his dry Ulster wit and limitless decency telling me: 'You'll be all right. The circuits have tripped. You should probably go in for a while …'

I do go into hospital, to a new locked ward, with the windows that don't open fully, and still signing out, and back in, when I go to the garden. I am grateful for the quiet, too tired to feel shame. That will come later, after the terror eases.

I know I should not have gone to Khartoum after the massacre. I hadn't stopped to think about the risk to my mind.

What is left is the rawness of a struggle with myself. *Who will I be?* The people who follow my journalism, by and large, are those who care about places torn apart by war or those labouring under injustice – a committed audience though not a vast one. *What will I do if I am not the person the audiences have always known?* This was the place into which my mind had fallen.

In the psychiatric hospital I keep to myself, apart from a few conversations in the TV room, and the nightly chats with nurses as they make their rounds. I find comfort in poetry, my old refuge, my prayer. In hospital I return to the writings of Edward Thomas. He was ravaged by depression. It set him apart from his family and followed him to war. He wrote to his wife Helen from the Western Front: 'I cannot think of ever being home again, and dare not think of never being there again.'[4] In 'The Owl', written after surviving the battles of 1915, he wrote of: 'What I escaped and others could not.'[5] Two years later, on 9 April 1917, he was killed in action.

I begin to write. This book is started as an attempt to understand myself, the first words written in the room above the adolescents' ward, interrupted by the nightly owls and the occasional traumas of a young woman downstairs, who screams at the nurses and batters the walls.

I start to see Cristina again. At our first meeting she takes out my bulky file. 'Since 2008, on and off, we've been meeting,' she says.

There is no judgement in her voice. It is a statement of fact.

'What am I going to do?'

'Let us first figure out what you are not going to do.'

Cristina makes me listen to the critical voices in my head, the ones that tell me I am nothing.

'Let's give the voices a name, the name of a person. Who will it be?'

I can think of a few. An old maths teacher at home, a long time ago, who regularly ridiculed my inability to grasp his subject. To me a nasty little man. The rugby coach who knew I was useless and didn't mind announcing it to everyone on the training pitch. But they come much later in my story. The feeling of nothingness came from a long way before. It was there in the chaos and unhappiness of my early years, in the baby who grew to a boy believing he was unlovable, because if he was lovable then his father would surely not be so unhappy or his mother either. All would have been peaceful if only he was lovable.

'There is no one person. It is people,' I say.

There is the pain inside me and the pain I have caused. This is the wellspring from which the critical voices come. When I quit drinking I followed the advice to keep things 'in the day'. No ruminating over the past or future. It worked for me then. When the voices start taunting, Cristina says, answer them with positive statements. But this is hard. Often in the past when somebody has said something kind about me as a person, I have felt moved in a way that has surprised them. *You are so grateful even for scraps of kindness.*

I start on a new anti-depressant. It does what they nearly always do. The savage anxiety ebbs away, everything flattens out. There is neither acute pain, nor anything you might call joy. Cristina and I work on practicalities. As a first step, I agree to arrange a meeting with the BBC on release from hospital and tell them I am stepping down from the job of Africa Editor. I will also tell them I will never again go to a place where I am in danger of being killed. It seems a simple rule; the complications around that statement I leave to a later date, as often before with my promises.

I will, however, still report on the consequences of war – on the refugees who are daily attempting to seek refuge in Europe; the broken political entities that emerge from war and how they in turn threaten the future peace; and on the trauma of war. I intend also to mount investigations into the crimes of war, after the fighting has ended. Of course this is still holding my hand close to the fire. I won't make myself a potential target. I will not witness actual killing and destruction but I'll still be meeting people who are traumatised by war and listening to their stories. This is as far as I am willing to allow myself to go in abstaining from war.

I leave hospital and take time off. I walk and I fish in Ireland. I ignore the news. I meet friends and go to AA meetings.

The pandemic comes and I am becalmed. The days of spring and summer are spent learning French and writing poetry. I get a dog, travelling one stormy day to the Welsh mountains to collect a Spanador (a Spaniel–Labrador cross) puppy called Deilo. The pup becomes my new therapist. He listens to me ramble on, and makes me walk every day with my grown-up children, a brown blur racing through the high grass along the Thames Path and through the fallen twigs and pine cones of 'Two-Storm Wood' in Richmond Park.

It is a constant motto of 12 Step fellowships that working on gratitude is an important prop to mental health. So, I make lists of what is good in my life. By any objective calculation I *should* be happy. I am still on anti-depressants because I am scared of being scared, scared too of getting angry with people and them thinking it would be better to leave me on my own. I am trying to only use Xanax if a big anxiety crisis hits, but the zolpidem is all that gets me to sleep at night. I know better than to proclaim myself healed. I am not.

Cristina says I need to face the ghosts of Rwanda. She believes avoidance is hindering my recovery. She wants me to have 'counter-narratives' of Rwanda to the ones that have brought me to my knees again and again.

'Find the good people in the stories of your past. Find them and see another Rwanda. See another Ukraine.'

'I am not going back to Rwanda.'

'Nobody is suggesting that. Just start working on your perceptions. Stop avoiding.'

I would probably have continued avoiding Rwanda. But somebody from the past intervened, and I could not turn away.

18

For Fear of a Dream

But anyway, I still believe I only sleep today,
That I'll wake up, a child again,
and start to laugh and play.

'Terezín', Michael Flack[1]

Before leaving London, I read as much as I can about the city in which she has settled. She has come here for love. Yet it is easy enough to see why Beata agreed with her husband to put down roots in Bordeaux. It is both elegant and intimate, a city by a broad river, the Garonne, which flows for 529 kilometres from the Spanish Pyrenees to the port of Bordeaux. It is a place of peace.

There is another hour before we meet. I am already in a state of apprehension. I sit in the drizzle near the market stalls of the Marché Saint Michel and read. As ever, I have with me several books of poetry. I try to force my mind to focus on the travails of *Huon of Bordeaux*, a knight who mistakenly kills the son of Emperor Charlemagne and is given a series of seemingly impossible tasks to complete if he wishes to live. One of Huon's companions has a dream of foreboding in which the knight's heart is ripped from his body by leopards; when he reveals it to Huon he is told: 'If by God we shall not return for fear of a dream, it would be forever our reproach and shame ...'[2]

I am struck by the line 'for fear of a dream'. What am I afraid of this rainy summer morning? The person I am meeting? Ridiculous. I already know her to be gentle and kind. She is the one who reached out first to me.

I am worried about how my visit will impact on her. The event that is bringing us together in Bordeaux took place nearly thirty years ago. The memory of the road we travelled brings a cold sweat. The eyes of the children gazing out from the interior of the truck. What they knew and what we knew. That country without illusions. How at any minute a choice could be made that would end in tragedy. Every minute of that journey was circumscribed. One drunk militiaman wielding a machete and we could have been thrown into a massacre. Or it might have come via an order from a soldier. As the *préfet* put it outside his office: there were 'no guarantees'. What would we have done if they tried to kill the children? Would I have been brave enough to try and intervene? In the end I did not have to make that choice. The children survived. She was among them, although I had no awareness of her presence at the time.

The house dates from the nineteenth century. It is situated on a side street in the old town near the wide river where later, after we've shared what remains to be told, we walk together in the afternoon rain.

Beata Umubyeyi Mairesse is a woman of grace and sensitivity. Her home is filled with books and quiet. There is art from Rwanda. She is an accomplished writer, and the author of a prize-winning novel and a collection of short stories.

Her eyes read my body language with a warm curiosity. She speaks softly and can appear reserved until something makes her laugh. Then she is transformed. The presence of a defiant lifeforce fills the kitchen. Beata says she is happy that I have come. For her this is part of a process, in which she tries to put the past into a reliable narrative.

Her boys, aged seven and thirteen, are upstairs doing their homework. They pop in briefly, shyly, and politely, before retreating to their studies.

Beata's husband, Yann, a physicist who works on research at the local university, makes us coffee and the three of us talk about the joys and challenges of raising children, especially in this age of social media, when hateful ideas spread like wildfire. I wonder how much she has shared with the boys about her experiences. 'We haven't been to Rwanda together yet,' she says, 'but I try the best I can with them … and little by little I'm going to give them books to read, and go there, show them that Rwanda is also a beautiful country with beautiful people, and it's not only the country where there was a genocide.'[3]

We begin to speak of those months between April and July 1994, when the ideology of extermination consumed the imaginations of huge numbers of Beata's fellow countrymen and women. She was fifteen when it began. Her father was Polish and her mother a Rwandan Tutsi. Her father, who has since died, left for Poland long before the genocide, but she is in contact with family there.

When the killings started, there was shooting and explosions. The night filled with screams and the whistles of the hunting gangs. Her mother knew enough of what Hutu mobs had done to Tutsis in the past to quickly pack a few belongings and find a place to hide. Beata recounts the story without tears, without faltering. Hers is not a narrative of horror, but of someone who believed she would survive, and needed to prepare for whatever came afterwards.

When the genocide began, she was at home with her mother in Butare:

We had to search for a place to hide, we had to take, you
know, stuff [as we] left the house, and when I talk with my
friends, who are survivors, they say: 'I took my favourite
dress', or some hadn't the time to take anything. But we had
that time and [instead of] my favourite toy I took my photo
album. I thought if I survive this is what I'm going to need. I
was already aware that what is important is you know the
memory, photos, pictures of the people of my life before, and
being able to prove that I have been to school, so I took my
diploma from school.[4]

After first hiding in their apartment, she and her mother found shelter in a cave. Even though friends had been killed, murdered in front of their parents, Beata was convinced that she would not die. They remained there for weeks until one day the murderers came. They killed two people who were hiding in the cave beside them. But when they came to the fifteen-year-old girl she struck an angry pose.

Beata is light-skinned. She decided to use her 'European' appearance to challenge the militia: 'I pretended to be angry at them saying: "Oh yes, I'm French, my father is French, and if you kill me the President of France is going to be mad at you. So, you don't have the right to kill me."'

As those of us who travelled in Rwanda at that time knew, the French were seen as allies by the genocidal regime. They had nurtured the government of the former president, Juvénal Habyarimana, long after they were aware of its extremist nature. In 1991 French troops joined the war against the guerrillas of the Tutsi-dominated Rwandan Patriotic Front, acting as advisors and, occasionally, taking part in combat operations. For all the killers knew, Beata and her mother might have been the family of a French businessman, soldier or official. The teenager argued for their lives and succeeded.

Eventually she and her mother made their way to the school where Alexis Briquet and his team from Terre des Hommes were preparing to evacuate hundreds of orphaned Tutsi children. The situation for mother and teenager was precarious. They should not have been there: according to the agreement reached between Terre des Hommes and the genocidal authorities, only orphaned children were allowed shelter. So even among the endangered Beata and her mother represented a different category, those for whom no exception, however tentative, had been made; those who could be killed on sight.

I do not remember seeing the mother and daughter when I looked inside the trucks that morning. This was of course intentional. They were lying flat, covered by blankets, with small children, some bandaged and bloodied, sitting on and around them.

Beata first contacted me about ten years after that journey. She emailed explaining that she had been on the convoy and asking if I had any video or photographs. I sent what I could find and put her in touch with other members of our BBC team. She came to London with her husband and we met briefly in a busy cafe on the South Bank. For days before her arrival, I was anxious and experiencing waves of sadness.

'You were crying,' she remembers. 'You didn't seem very well. I saw it, and then, and then at that moment I thought: "Okay, my coming here is very hard for him, and that maybe he's not ready for that." But at the same time you seemed happy to see me, and also crying. I didn't insist on talking a lot. I was asking you to go back in, I didn't realise that you were somehow stuck there. I thought this is not the right moment. Maybe this time will come.'

Now I was with her, responding to her message to get in touch. Beata had more questions about the journey. She was researching the life of Alexis Briquet who had died earlier in the year from cancer. She'd also traced many other children who had been on the convoy:

> Some sent very beautiful messages when I told them Alex was dying, saying 'We are the children of the convoy. You saved our lives', and thanking him. Some were not ready for that, were not ready to go back in that story. And I think they have a kind of trauma, even if some think that everything is all right now. But I think having this memory somewhere I will keep it for them, and one day, if they want to go back there, they will find it, because otherwise everything disappears.[5]

She spoke with Alexis on the phone a few times before he passed away and thanked him for saving her life and that of her mother. There was more to it than thanking him though. I think she may have been looking for proof that she had not imagined it all, that it had really happened. Too often people who had not been there would talk about the genocide as something 'unspeakable'. Reaching out to the other survivors helped her to place the experiences of 1994 in a place of reality. 'I think there's nothing worse than living through something like that, and being the only one, not having anybody to share this with.'

She is still searching for other children of that convoy. There were many more than she has been able to trace so far.

After arriving as a refugee in France in 1994, Beata was placed with a French family whose daughter was suffering from schizophrenia. 'I was lucky when I arrived in France. The family were very much aware of mental health issues.' It is not likely she would have been able to face the past in this way without the help of therapy. 'They immediately told me you must go and see a shrink,' she continues. 'So, since then I've been seeing shrinks. I started taking care of my mental health. It was not only about the genocide. It was also about my personal life, my family's history, and all those things ... I'm still working on it. It's a lifelong journey ...'

There will be sadness when April comes, the date when the genocide began. She will give this pain its space. She may cry. But it will not take over her life. Pain is like a wild animal to be tamed, Beata explains. You learn to not allow yourself to be invaded, but to invite it at a time of your choosing. Trying to erase the pain is like erasing part of yourself.

Listening to her reasoned explanation I see how she has taken the awfulness of her memories and shaped them into a monument against the denial of genocide. But she also uses them as a spur to embrace the beauty in life. I am learning as I listen. In the last few years, she has trained in mental health and runs a suicide prevention programme in Bordeaux.

'I have always been fighting against death in different ways,' she says. Her work – to preserve memory, to help other survivors, to help the suicidally depressed – is an act of love.

We walk to the river on our way to have lunch. It is raining but nothing like the downpours of Rwanda whose volume obliterated all other noise. A hawk floats above the water and Beata explains that falcons are the totem of her clan.

She is preparing for a reunion with some of the Terre des Hommes staff, including Deanna, Alexis Briquet's wife, in a few months' time. She asks if I would like to come. I say I will think about it. But I feel that as a journalist I might change the experience for the others, perhaps make them uneasy, no matter how much I try to avoid doing so. There is, too, the old doubt: I am not worthy of being with them. What have I suffered by comparison?

We talk of her 'beautiful things' in life, like music and poetry – especially poetry. Beata recalls a poem by the French Auschwitz

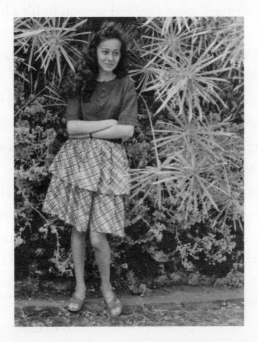

Beata Umubyeyi Mairesse as a teenager. Her generosity and grace have helped me so much. (*Beata Umubyeyi Mairesse*)

survivor Charlotte Delbo, whose husband was executed in the camp.

> Learn to walk and to laugh
> Because it would be too senseless
> After all
> For so many to have died
> While you live
> Doing nothing with your life.[6]

Beata still dreams of Rwanda. Two or three times a week. But they are not dreams of genocide. Instead, her subconscious mind goes back to the world before the slaughter. Everyday scenes in lush green and sunlight.

The dead of her Rwanda cannot be brought back. The dead I saw cannot be unseen. But what a waste it would be to have witnessed all that, she says, and not have made our own lives as happy as we can.

Point taken, I say.

She writes to me a few days later asking how I am. I say I am much better for having seen her. We agree to meet with our loved ones in the summer.

When I think of Rwanda now, I will try to replace the dead with the image of Beata and her husband and boys. The picture of life.

19

Gathering In

And so it was I entered the broken world,
To trace the visionary company of love, its voice
An instant in the wind ...
... And through whose pulse I hear, counting the strokes
My veins recall and add, revived and sure
The angelus of wars my chest evokes:
What I hold healed, original now, and pure ...

'The Broken Tower', Hart Crane[1]

It is the spring of 2021 and I have not been to a battlefield in two years. But I have made history programmes and I've commentated live on the anniversaries of D Day, VJ Day, and Remembrance Sunday. There have been journeys to European frontiers where border guards beat back those fleeing poverty and war. I have gone into the pandemic emergency wards, carefully kitted out in PPE, to report on the courage of NHS workers, and to remote villages in England to tell the stories of communities supporting their elderly and disabled neighbours. I have felt no threat. My PTSD symptoms are still present, especially the hyper-vigilance, but they are milder. The Rwandan nightmares have stopped.

The nearest I come to drama is when my car becomes snow-bound on a mountain in Derbyshire. I am rescued by a British Indian doctor who has brought his family to live here to escape the claustrophobia of London.

I find myself seeking narratives that reflect the better angels of human nature. I cannot say that I miss war. But I do yearn to visit my friend the beekeeper and his wife in Ukraine. I wonder if they had stayed in Piski under the constant exchanges of fire, and I think too about their mental welfare, after surviving so long in that embattled place.

I see now that this revisiting of people I have come to care about, is also a means of reassurance. To find that they are well gives me strength to have faith in my own journey.

I call Daryna in Kyiv and ask her to see if Anatoly and Svetlana Kosse are still living in Piski. If so, then a visit will be out of the question. The village is still right on the line of contact between the two armies. But she calls back a day later to say that they have moved to the peaceful village of Kolmar, about a hundred kilo-metres away from Piski and the fighting.

'They would be delighted to see us,' Daryna continues.

Going to Ukraine feels like a liberation. The age of Covid has closed borders over the previous eighteen months, but now I can travel again. Six years after our first meeting I am on my way back to see Anatoly and Svetlana.

In a car park on the banks of the Dnieper on an evening of warm spring light I am reunited with Daryna and Sasha. Such joy we feel in each other's company. After he heard I got the Africa job Sasha wondered if we would ever see each other again. 'I was told you had gone to Africa and thought you would forget us,' he chides.

Never, I reassure him, never would I forget.

He tells me his son is married with a child of his own. *Grandfather Sasha!* I say. That night over dinner we talk about our adventures in the Donbas. I remind him of the day at the Ukrainian checkpoint outside Mariupol, when a big mine went off and how our hearts jumped into our mouths but then Sasha had reversed at speed – no turning on the narrow road where mines might have been set – and got us out of danger and back to the city, as so many times before.

After dinner, Daryna asks to speak to me away from the others. She appears nervous. 'I am leaving the BBC,' she says. The news comes as a surprise. She is highly valued, immensely capable. As she spells out her reasons, I try to persuade her to stay. But I know it is pointless. I know that the war has taken away her home in Donetsk and there would be no going back any time soon. Putin's stooges in the east have put her on a blacklist. Return would mean arrest and probable disappearance into one of the grim jails of the puppet regime.

When war broke out in eastern Ukraine, Daryna was working as a translator for businesses. She was also a single mother whose extended family of mother, brother and sister depended on her for financial support. Within weeks of the conflict starting, she found herself in the middle of firefights. She witnessed dogs ravaging corpses. She saw her home city become a hellhole where the rule of law disappeared.

After moving her young son, her mother and brother and sister to Kyiv, she tried to build a new life in the capital. There was no war there and her son went to a good school. She met a man who was kind to her and to the boy. Daryna knew he had been caught in the deadly ambush at Ilovaisk in August 2014, when Ukrainian volunteers were massacred after being promised safe passage by the Russian proxies. Surrounded at their base in a school, the men and women of the volunteer battalion came under relentless rocket and shell fire. Those who tried to drive out in a convoy were blasted by tanks. Medical supplies for the wounded were derisory. One medic reported trying to stanch severe wounds with tampons.

He was one of those who crawled out by night and made his way across enemy territory before reaching the Ukrainian lines, a gruelling cross-country journey. In the end the burden of his PTSD pushed them apart. She could understand his suffering, but she could not cure it.

Trauma is everywhere in Ukraine, but most acute among the veterans, the civilians living in the embattled eastern zone, and the local journalists covering the war week in and week out. In the spring of 2021, Putin threatens escalation. Most people I meet worry about a bigger Russian attack, one that might not stop in the Donbas but go all the way to Kyiv.

I wish Daryna well and ask that we stay friends. I need not worry, she says. The friendships made in war zones have a habit of enduring.

There is no Richard Stacey, the man with whom we made the first journeys to the Donbas. We are not going to go to the front lines, and therefore do not need a security advisor. But even if we were he would not have been available. Late last year he called to say that a tumour had been found next to his brain. It was too dangerous to operate but the doctors were going to try chemo and radiotherapy. The growth would kill him, eventually, they said, but they wanted to give him as much time as possible. Rich sent a note: 'I won't be getting away from this firefight I'm afraid … I'll fight this is as long as I can. I just wanted to update my friends who I've been [with] in some of the most difficult situations and it has never fazed me at all. But now I am facing something that is taking me away and I can't control it ... Give my love to Daryna.'[2]

I missed him here, even if there was no danger where we were going. I missed the sanity and the willingness to call me out when he thought I was talking bullshit. I missed the kindness.

A good man was dying.

We set off for the beekeeper's place at dawn, into the familiar landscape of corn and sunflower fields, heading east towards the line of contact but, emphatically, not anywhere near the fighting.

I am in the company of good people, and I am going to meet friends. I have not seen them in five years. They are survivors of war *and* the pandemic. Ukraine's vaccination rates are deplorably low – only 30 per cent of the population – but Anatoly and Svetlana have managed to get their injections.

The couple moved here two years before, after the army made Piski a closed military zone. There had been a series of crises. Several nearby houses were struck by shells. Their own windows were blown out. At some point soon, they feared, there would be a direct hit, or one close enough to kill. A neighbour who had moved to Kolmar told them there was a dilapidated house for sale. They could buy it cheaply with their savings and start a new life. Both were now seventy-four years of age. I wondered what kind of a new life would they find after a lifetime in Piski?

We arrive in Kolmar to find the place almost deserted. There is patriotic music playing from a marquee in front of the town hall. 'It is Independence Day,' Daryna explains. A few men are sitting drinking in a garden facing the square, bored, not bothering to watch as we drive past. We turn down a rutted lane and I see a familiar figure standing by the roadside.

The beekeeper waves, and as we draw closer, I see his broad smile. He calls out to Svetlana in the garden that we're here.

No drug could give me the joy I feel in their embrace. Svetlana too has tears of merriment in her eyes as she laughs. They have brought to their new home the steel garden gate, with the shrapnel marks, I remember from our first visit to Piski. But that is the only memento of war. Their garden here is in its first bloom of flowers and herbs, even small vines for their homemade wine, and drills where they have planted potatoes, beans, and carrots. Life is flourishing in this small patch of land.

Anatoly brought with him his bees from Piski, but they died within a few weeks, killed by the pesticide a local farmer had sprayed on his land and hedgerows. Now Anatoly has a new colony and his bees are working the flowers. They are already producing honey.

We go inside for lunch. The kitchen table is crowded with food: roast pork covered in melted cheese, beet salad, mashed potato, pickles, horseradish, a jar of plum kompot – the sweet juice to balance the salty pickles. As if we'd never been away.

When I ask what happened to make them leave Piski, Svetlana speaks of the shelling and the health problems that were creeping up on them both. They struggled to sleep. Svetlana said her nerves had become strained, wondering when their luck would run out, and Anatoly was having heart problems. 'So, when the neighbour who had left for Kolmar called and asked: "Are you going to wait for the next one to hit you?" we decided to go.'[3]

Anatoly describes meeting an officer in the laneway outside their house who was transporting the corpses of three soldiers who had been killed that day. 'He asked me: "What shall I say to their children – all of them have kids?" Those kids were left with no father. Do they need this war? Who needs this war?'[4]

Svetlana's father fought through the Second World War 'from Zaporizhia to Berlin and Prague' and was awarded the Red Star for courage in battle. 'He went through that war for four years. But it was *just* four years. Here we are in our seventh year of the war. I have high blood pressure. My back and arms are sore, and my nerves are hurting. Who needs this?'[5]

It was an agony to wrench themselves away from the Piski house, they say, leaving the place where Svetlana had grown up and where they had spent fifty years of married life and raised two daughters. But 'it is not about a house. We were expecting grand-children, and as grandchildren are usually spending summers in a village, we bought special types of strawberries, apricots and lots of other plants for our garden … and now we are here and have to start everything from the beginning again.'[6]

Sometimes Svetlana dreams she is back in the old house and her parents are there. When she wakes, she remembers the news from Piski, what they have been told by soldiers they know. 'Everything is ruined or burned, only chimneys are left and stick-ing out. Our house burned down. There is no roof.'[7]

A sadness has settled around the table. I ask about the old woman, Sonya Tolmachova, and her disabled son. They are still there, says Svetlana, because there is nowhere to send them where they can be together, so the military turn a blind eye to their pres-ence. The previous year Sonya was taken to hospital after a bad fall and her boy sent to an institution. He was distraught without his mother and when she recovered they made their way back through the barbed wire, and around the minefield and into their home. Soldiers brought them food. They see nobody. They are waiting for the war to end.

For all the pity in the stories they tell, Anatoly and Svetlana are fundamentally happy. Everything around them is broken but they have stayed solid. I ask a naive question, but the only one that seems to matter in the circumstances: 'What is the secret of being happy?'

Anatoly begins to laugh.

'Who would not be happy with such a mischievous wife?' He leans his head towards Svetlana. She begins to sing a song from long ago in their courtship: '*The best gift for me is you. Is you …* *Is you …*' Love is his answer to my question. It's like a favourite line of mine from Raymond Carver, where he describes loving the music rivers make, 'loving everything that increases me',[8] and like Beata back at the river in Bordeaux and hearing her injunction to live for the good in life because it is what we owe to the dead.

We go back outside to the hives. Anatoly produces a can of smoke to calm the bees. He lifts a frame from the hive, revealing a mass of working creatures, and speaks to them with gentleness. '*It's okay my little sweeties … We have to clean this.*'

A bee lands on his right hand.

'I just like to take care of them,' he says. 'Here is one bee I took. It is just one of ten thousand. It is not that important on its own, but I feel sorry for it, it is so tiny.'

There is, in this house, as there had been in their first house in Piski, a tenacious humanity fighting to overcome the cruelties of war. It is not that Anatoly and Svetlana are impervious to pain. But life has equipped them – through their happy childhoods, the fortunes of a long peace in the old imperium, and the match of their personalities – with the strength equal to the challenges of this troubled new world. The generosity they show to others brought its own reward when they were displaced. There was the neighbour who found them the house in Kolmar, the friends who regularly call to see how they are settling in. They are cherished by a community that has maintained its ties despite being uprooted by war.

I begin to feel drowsy, the effects of the early start and the abundant lunch. Svetlana tells me to go inside and lie on a couch in the sitting room. They will wake me for coffee in an hour. I do as I am told and drowse off to the sound of their chatter beyond the window. In the past I have felt sadness when saying goodbye to them. This time it is different. They are safe here. But there is another reason for the absence of that melancholy which marked previous departures. In that moment I feel truly as if I have left the wars. We part believing that the strain of life on the front line is behind us all.

On our way back to Kyiv I asked Daryna if she would change her mind about leaving. 'No, I will find another life. Maybe I will travel.' There is an unassailable logic to her decision, and I do not have it in my heart to try and persuade her otherwise. Although the threat from Putin's army feels as if it has dissipated, the war could escalate again and if she stays, she might feel the journalist's urge to deploy.

Daryna doesn't want to impose a burden of worry on her son. Like her I feel guilty for the anxiety my troubles have caused to loved ones. But guilt is also a trap. If I feel self-loathing I start to need to escape to war, the ultimate land of forgetting. Enough is enough.

There is much that I have messed up but ruminating on that will sink me. I am weary from PTSD. I cannot bear the idea of another breakdown, the sense of failure that it will bring. I think of a message sent to me by an old friend, a girl I had loved as a teenaged boy, and whose family had offered me refuge from the trauma of childhood. She remains dear in my memory. 'If anyone I know deserves peace of mind, you do,' she wrote. I was so grateful to hear that from someone who knew the place I had come from.

The voice that tells me I am worthless, and which drove me from one war to another, is a voice I recognise as my own. Peace of mind, if it is to come, will only arrive at my own beckoning.

Epilogue
Kinder Voices

Lviv, Western Ukraine, March 2022

Even when the spring sunlight fills the little park it remains an unsettling place. The Jewish world commemorated at Arsenalna Square was destroyed by genocide: the people who worshipped at the Golden Rose synagogue were either exiled or killed. There is no escape from history here. It is present in the memorial stones for the dead and in the void left by a murdered generation.

The past collides with the present in other ways too. You can hear it in the rattle of today's refugee suitcases being pulled across the same cobblestoned streets where, in the high summer of 1941, the Germans and their Ukrainian collaborators chased Jews to their deaths. The photos of those days are some of the most terrible of the Holocaust: women being stripped and beaten before jeering mobs; eyes wide in horror, mouths frozen in mid-scream.

I am here because on 24 February 2022, Vladimir Putin's armies attacked Ukraine. I was asleep in London when the first missiles landed in Kyiv and the airborne forces attacked Hostomel airport, a huge cargo and aircraft testing centre in the city's suburbs. Four days previously I had flown out of Kyiv to avoid the looming invasion. The battle with myself, between the addict who wanted to stay and the other person, trying to be better, was settled by picking up a phone and booking a flight, one of the last as it turned out, back to London.

I had become convinced in the previous weeks that a Russian attack was imminent, arguing over dinner with colleagues that Putin would do so because he judged the world to be a cynical place where the Western powers would abandon Ukraine to its fate, just as they had left the Syrians and Afghans to the mercy of their tormentors. So it came to pass, at least as far as his decision-making process was concerned. Putin was a bully who judged his enemies to be weak, whose psychology was that of a paranoid street thug, and who listened only to the words of flattering and fearful subordinates whose position and wealth depended entirely on his whim. He turned out to be wrong, however, in his estimation of the Western response.

On the morning of the invasion, I was woken at home by a message from the news desk: 'He's done it. Can you do the refugee story?' Others were already in or were heading to the combat zone. I would not be going where there was any fighting. That was the deal.

Thousands of people were on the move towards Ukraine's western borders, most obviously the frontier with Poland. The fighting was taking place 600 kilometres to the east, around Kyiv and further east again at Kharkiv and the cities of the Donbas, and around Kherson on the Black Sea, and south-east at Mariupol on the Sea of Azov. I knew all of these places well, and I knew the devastating power of artillery. I did not need to work hard to imagine how the attackers were obliterating homes and lives.

Daryna called. She was in tears. No matter how much she had anticipated the possibility of an invasion, now that it had happened she was in shock. Worse, she was not at home in Kyiv but on a business trip to Spain. Her precious son was with his grandmother in the capital and there was no way of reaching them. I tried to console her and advised on routes out to Europe for her mother and son.

By the following evening I was crossing from Poland into Ukraine. We went by foot over the frontier, myself and producer Alice Doyard and cameraman Nik Millard. Alice had been with me down many other challenging roads in Africa and on the refugee trail in Europe, and I had covered the Kosovo crisis with Nik, whose kindness I remembered well in those days in Kukës when I was struggling in the final phase of my drinking. I was with good people.

It was quiet on the Polish side. We pushed our trolley of luggage up the hill, past the nervy Ukrainian guards and into chaos. Thousands of people were massing to cross and behind them, already fleeing the east and south, were millions more. A line of

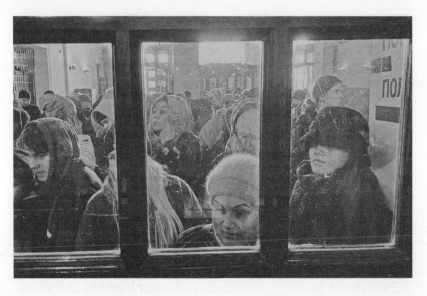

Refugees waiting for a train at Lviv station.

cars stretched forty kilometres in the direction of Lviv. A woman was giving birth on the side of the road. Children wailed. Most people seemed to have brought their pets. The cats and dogs, and a solitary rabbit, gave the whole scene an air of domesticity – a desperate domesticity, the animals one of the few mobile parts of the secure world that was being lost with every shuffle forward to the frontier. All of society was here, bar the men of fighting age, partners, husbands, brothers, sons, who were obliged by law to stay.

I switched to professional mode. I focused on telling the stories of the people we encountered but, with Cristina's words in mind, I tried to do so with a self-protective distance. *Repeat to yourself: I am not responsible. I cannot help everybody. I am not here to rescue anyone. Tell the story, don't get swallowed by it.*

There were moments when I felt tears coming: watching people fight each other to board trains in the first days of the war; the elderly woman from the bombed theatre in Mariupol, her pale, frightened face covered in bruises; the sight of a father's palm pressed against a windowpane, all those fathers we saw in the moments of farewell.

Left to their own devices I knew these feelings would come back and hurt me later on. Before leaving home I had set in place a routine of 'psychological hygiene'. Each night our team shared what we felt about the things we had seen – a kind of mobile therapy that allowed feelings to be expressed there and then without the build-up that could lead to any of us being overwhelmed. I also asked Cristina if she and I could do regular therapy on Zoom, and I made the time, no matter what else was happening, to keep the appointments. There were moments that triggered deep fear: the howls of air-raid sirens erupting several times a day and sometimes in the middle of the night.

I tried to reach Anatoly and Svetlana in Kolmar but their phones were not ringing. I scan the crowds at Lviv station for their faces, thinking they might have joined the great exodus to the west. After three or four days we manage to make contact: Anatoly is at home, and Svetlana is in hospital recovering from Covid. He is sure she will be well soon, but they are not going to move, even though the Russians could easily come their way. I think of him alone, listening to the news of the war, wondering when this woman he adores will be released from hospital, and praying that they will not be uprooted once more.

I think of them every time I hear armchair experts talk about a 'new security architecture for Europe', debating Ukraine as a 'sphere of influence', as if the lives of its people are some possession that can be parcelled out between the great powers. Anatoly and Svetlana, these makers of good bread and honey, are worth more than that.

If there is likely to be a threat to my emotional stability in Ukraine now it will come not from imminent physical danger but from 'moral injury', the hardest wound to heal because the war being what it is, the injustices keep multiplying, the ones we see and report, and the countless others we do not. In these days of late February I fear the emotional hangover that will come if Putin quickly takes Kyiv, and Ukraine becomes a vassal state ruled by his puppets. I am not naive about the limitations of governance in Zelensky's Ukraine, but it is a better place by far than the oligarchy of the pro-Putin era before the revolution of 2014.

In Lviv, I am surrounded by idealistic young people volunteering to serve their country. They pack food and clothing for people in the east. The station becomes a vast hub of volunteers who help every family fleeing west. There is music at night for the refugees, who huddle around braziers before catching the early morning trains. I am constantly witnessing the expression of human decency.

Though I am utterly powerless to influence any of what is happening, I still worry. Will the West abandon Ukraine as it abandoned the Rwandan Tutsis in 1994, or the Afghans in 2021? But there is a big difference between Rwanda and Ukraine. Rwanda did not count for the powerful nations of the world. It was a place they felt they could safely ignore. But Ukraine matters politically to Washington and Brussels and London. It is a front line on the doorstep of the Western world. A charismatic president is rallying his people. The world's media is here to report the country's fight.

There are moments when my addictive impulse surges, and one in particular when I might have walked back into the line of fire and upended my chances of recovery. I suggest to London that we make a short film about the train journey from Lviv to Kyiv, and back again: the story of the railways and how they keep running through the Russian invasion is emblematic of the Ukrainian struggle as a whole. Trains brave attack to carry refugees, soldiers, food, weapons, and the foreign political leaders brave enough to make the journey to see President Zelensky. The railways people say yes to the trip. I begin to bargain with myself and rehearse my arguments to the BBC.

I will stay on the train and in railway stations. They have very good alarm systems to warn of attack ...

Yes, but what happens if they bomb the track, the train, or the stations?

It's highly unlikely. They have largely avoided attack so far [this would change]. *The train would be blacked out to avoid presenting a target.*

280

I speak to my editor. 'I don't really think it's a good idea, do you?' he says. There is a pause. I am embarrassed, as if I've been caught out, like somebody way back smelling my breath to see if I have been drinking.

I admit, without a struggle, that it is not a good idea. The rest of the crew can go without me if they want. After being stuck in Lviv for three weeks they jump at the chance. I see them off as they board the train west, with aid workers and soldiers, late at night. I feel guilty to have them go without me, but there are also feelings of envy. I mention to Alice that the piece might be more 'powerful' if I go with them, travelling through the night.

'Really?' she replies. 'The piece will be just as good either way.' From a place of care and kindness, she is telling me: *Get over yourself. It isn't worth the risk to your mind. Your 'hero' days are over. Your journalism isn't indispensable, but your life is. Staying here on the platform is the stronger thing. Do it for yourself.*

I am briefly frustrated, but my feet are standing where they should be.

I still get angry over things that would not trouble most people. I am not cured of PTSD. I am learning to live with it. My insecurities can still start me bargaining with myself about what is safe and what is not. Sometimes I fight that hour by hour. But I've kept to the 'no combat' part of my promise. Maybe that part will get easier, the urge will die away, the way it became second nature not to drink when I kept doing the work of sobriety.

I still jump when a plate falls or a car backfires. Some mornings my T-shirt and the pillow are soaking wet after a bad night. In the mornings I barely remember my dreams, but I know I have been visited. Recently I woke up to the sound of a massive explosion outside the building, and then I realised the missile had landed in a dream, and I was safe.

Being well requires work: keep talking to Cristina, to others recovering from PTSD. Say no every time the urge comes into my mind. Each night I sit and write my gratitude list, as I was taught back in rehab. I am sober. I can be depended on to turn up when I promise, to be a reassuring voice on the other end of the phone for those I love, at any time of the day or night, to be a true friend. I am loved. I don't feel lost. As I write I have been two months off anti-depressants. I am sleeping without the aid of any pills. I have not turned to Xanax to fight my anxiety in over six months. This makes me feel proud. I am done with promises, except to say I will do my best, and I will try to listen to the kinder voices. They are many and bright.

A Note on Sources

This book is the result of many sources and inspirations. I have leaned heavily on the memories of colleagues and friends who were with me at various stages of the journey. Among those who read the manuscript and gave feedback were Rizwana Hamid, Fred Scott, Greg Marinovich, Beata Umubyeyi Mairesse, Daryna Meyer and Eugene McVeigh. Chris Cleave, novelist and psycho-therapist, was always on hand to offer considered reflections.

On the therapeutic front I am indebted to Dr Niall Campbell and Cristina Garcia Llavona for their insights on PTSD, and to Dr Tony Humphreys of Cork for his early observations on child-hood trauma and abandonment. Professor Simon Wessely of King's College London gave me valuable advice on trauma and family history.

To Paul Barrett in London and Patrick Brown on Pender Island, British Columbia, many thanks for your advice over the years on the connections between addiction and PTSD.

I have once again made generous use of the files available at both the Military Archives in Dublin and the National Archives at Kew Gardens. The archivists in both places have my lasting gratitude.

On the topic of the Great Famine I was lucky to be able to refer to the exceptional work of Bryan MacMahon (*The Great Famine in Tralee and North Kerry*, Mercier Press, 2017) and John D. Pierse (*Teampall Bán and Aspects of the Famine in North Kerry*, Listowel Tidy Towns Committee, 2014). Cathal Póirtér's oral history of the period (*Famine Echoes*, Gill and Macmillan, 2015) provided essential context of the lived experience of the hunger. For an understanding of the larger social and psychological issues of this period I recommend the works of Professor Cormac O'Gráda, Professor Emeritus of Economics, University College Dublin, and Professor Brendan Kelly (*The History of Psychiatry in Ireland*, Irish Academic Press, 2016).

In looking into trauma and the Irish Revolution I was given generous help by Professor Linda Connolly of Maynooth University who read a draft of the chapters on my grandmother, and by Andy Bielenberg, University College Cork, and Sean William Gannon, Trinity College Dublin, who helped me to investigate the life of William Darcy. I was also inspired by the work of Síobhra Aiken (*Spiritual Wounds: Trauma, Testimony and the Irish Civil War*, Irish Academic Press, 2022).

Although there is a growing body of literature on PTSD, the study of war journalists and trauma is still at a relatively early stage. I would refer those interested in learning more to the work of Professor Anthony Feinstein of the University of Toronto and to the DART Trauma Center at Columbia University, New York, https://dartcenter.org

I am grateful for the insight and challenges offered in the work of the late Susan Sontag (*Regarding the Pain of Others*, Penguin, 2003) and to Lindsey Hilsum (*In Extremis: The Life of War Correspondent Marie Colvin*, Chatto and Windus, 2018) and Clare Campbell (*Out of It*, Hodder, 2008).

I have also been helped personally and professionally by the work of the following authors: Bessel van der Kolk (*The Body*

Keeps the Score: Mind, Brain and Body in the Transformation of Trauma, Penguin, 2014), Janet Geringer Woititz (*Adult Children of Alcoholics at Home, at Work and in Love*, Health Communications Inc., 2002), Meg Jay (*Supernormal: Childhood Adversity and the Untold Story of Resilience*, Canongate, 2018).

I have also drawn from a substantial number of online sources which are acknowledged in the endnotes. One of the great advantages of the internet age is the availability of a wide range of research materials at the touch of a keyboard.

My thanks are due to Maxime Mojon-Doyard who has given vital assistance in clearing copyright permissions. All efforts have been made to seek clearance. Where it has not been possible any omissions that are pointed out will be corrected in future editions.

This book is a chronicle of pain, not only mine. In order to respect privacy I have not identified all of the people I encountered, or who accompanied me, at different stages on the journey through addiction and post-traumatic stress disorder. For the same reason on a small number of occasions I have excluded certain potentially identifying geographical or personal details.

I am grateful to Curtis Brown Group Ltd, London on behalf of the Beneficiaries of The Estate of Stephen Spender for permission to quote from 'The War God', copyright © Stephen Spender 1933.

Acknowledgements

Thank you to the many who helped see me this far. They are loved ones, friends, colleagues, people who are close to me, and those who hardly knew me but stopped to be kind.

I thank my beautiful children Daniel and Holly, my life's greatest and most enduring gifts, and their mother Anne, for their great compassion and support.

My family – the Keanes, Hassetts, Purtills, O'Connors, Schusters, Klabens, O'Sheas – have been telling me stories for years and listening to mine with great tolerance and undying loyalty. Mo ghrá dhaoibh go léir.

Arabella Pike has the greatest quality an editor can bring: the courage to back her authors, no matter how difficult the subject. She is a constant inspiration. Over the years Arabella and her team at William Collins, Kate Johnson and Iain Hunt, have steered my books to publication with creativity and patience.

Thank you also to my agent Peter Straus and his team at Rogers, Coleridge and White for their calm and focused help.

Gratitude also to Mike Connolly, Andy Dunne, Elsa Hunter-Weston, Martha O'Kane and Rachel Hooper – the team behind the BBC documentary *Living with PTSD* – as well as the staff and clients of the WAVE Trauma Centre in Belfast, for their openness and welcome. Sarah Ward Lilley at the BBC was an early initiator of trauma support for staff and was endlessly kind and supportive to me.

Dr Conor Brosnan, Jack Ahern and Dr Mary McAuliffe in Listowel gave generously of their time and knowledge. Bill and Denise Whelan in Connemara and New York provided the warmth that drove the journey on when I had my doubts.

Over the years I have been fortunate to work as part of some exceptional teams in the field. Thank you in particular to Milton Nkosi, Tony Fallshaw, Nik Millard, David McIlveen, Darren Conway, Glenn Middleton, Hamilton Wende, David Harrison, Mike Robinson, Katherine Quarmby, Kate Benyon-Tinker, Fiona Anderson, Thea Guest, Piers Scholfield, Richard Stacey, Ian Watt, Kevin Sissons and Kevin Sweeney – all of them the very best of the best.

To Alice Doyard I owe a continuing debt of gratitude. For the insights of a thoughtful teller of traumatic stories, the kindness of a great human being, and the welcome and hospitality of the Doyard clan.

Finally thank you to my mother, Maura, for her shining example of perseverance, whatever the weather, and to my late father, Eamonn, who kept trying to be the best man he could.

Notes

Prologue: A Trail of Shadows

1. Suzanne Moore, *Guardian*, 27 January 2020.
2. Cristina Garcia-Llavona, interview with author, 2020.
3. Sheridan Le Fanu, *Green Tea*, London, 1872.
4. Carl Jung, *The Undiscovered Self*, London, 1958.
5. A. Feinstein, J. Owen, and N. Blair, 'A Hazardous Profession: War, Journalists, and Psychopathology', *American Journal of Psychiatry*, Vol. 159, 9, 2002.
6. Claudia J. Dewane, 'The Legacy of Addictions: A Form of Complex PTSD?', *Social Work Today*, Vol. 10, No. 6, December 2010, p. 16.

Chapter 1: The Lying Mirror

1. Edward Thomas, *Selected Poems*, ed. Matthew Hollis, London, 2011.
2. Anton Chekhov, 'Perpetuum Mobile', *The Unknown Chekhov and Other Writings*, trans. of 1884 version by Avrahm Yarmolinsky, Ecco, New York, 1954.
3. Samuel Taylor Coleridge, The Rime of the Ancient Mariner, 1834 edition online, Perfection Learning Corporation, 2000.

Chapter 2: Shapings

1. Sara Teasdale, 'Fear', *The Collected Poems of Sara Teasdale*, Pantianos Classics, 2017, p. 48.
2. Percy French, 'The Mountains of Mourne', *c.*1896.
3. Maya Opendak and Regina M. Sullivan, *Unique infant neurobiology produces distinctive trauma processing*, Elsevier Publishing, https://doi.org/1016/j.dcn.2019.100637

4. National Scientific Council on the Developing Child. 2005/2014, *Excessive Stress Disrupts the Architecture of the Developing Brain: Working Paper 3*; updated edition: http://www.developingchild.harvard.edu
5. J. M. Synge, *The Playboy of the Western World*, 1907.
6. Evan Boland, 'Domestic Violence', William Norton and Company, 2007.
7. Reverend Father Thomas, *Summarised Life of the Great Temperance Apostle Father Theobald Matthew*, Guy and Co., Cork, 1902.
8. Claudine Rankine, from *Citizen – An American Lyric*, Penguin Books, 2014, p. 89.
9. www.stmichaelscollege.ie
10. John B. Keane, *Self Portrait*, Mercier Press, 1964, p. 15.
11. Moira J. Maguire, 'The Punishment and Abuse of Children in Twentieth Century Ireland', *Journal of Social History*, Vol. 38, Issue 3, Spring 2005, pp. 635–52, https://doi.org/10.1353/jsh.2005.0023
12. 'Anger and Trauma', US Department of Veterans Affairs: https://www.ptsd.va.gov/understand/related/anger.asp
13. Dr Janet Woititz, *Adult Children of Alcoholics*, Health Communications, Inc., Florida, 1983, p. 21.
14. Thomas Hardy, *The Mayor of Casterbridge*, 1886, London, Project Gutenberg edn, Kindle, Chapter 45, p. 745.
15. 'Priest gets suspended term for sex assaults on students', *Irish Times*, 20 March 2009.
16. Ibid.
17. John Boyne, interviewed by Cahir O'Doherty in the *Irish Voice*, 10 February 2015.
18. Gemma O'Doherty, 'Terror Nure', *Village Magazine*, 21 December 2017.

Chapter 3: Generations Fighting

1. Javier Ceras, *Lord of All the Dead*, London, 2020, MacLehose Press, pp. 312–13.
2. William Steuart Trench, *Realities of Irish Life*, Dublin, 1868, p. 120.
3. Ibid.
4. Samuel Lewis, *A Topographical Dictionary of Ireland*, S. Lewis, London, 1837.
5. William Carleton, *The Black Prophet*, Collier, New York, 1881, Project Gutenberg edition, 2005.
6. *Limerick and Clare Examiner*, 1847, cited in Senan Scanlon, 'Vandeleurs in Kilrush, County Clare', Clare County Library, https://www.clarelibrary.ie/eolas/coclare/genealogy/don_tran/fam_his/vandeleurs/famine.htm

7. Douglas Hyde, cited in Rosa Gonzaléz, 'The Unappeasable Hunger for Land', *Revista Alicantina de Estudios Ingleses* 5 (1992): 84.
8. Cormac O'Gráda, 'Famine, Trauma and Memory', *Folklore Journal of Ireland*, Bealoideas, 69: 121–43, http://hdl.handle.net/10197/455, 2001.
9. Cathal Póirtéir, *Famine Echoes: An Oral History of Ireland's Greatest Tragedy*, Gill and MacMillan, Dublin, 1995, Kindle edn, location 1544.
10. Michael Hartnett, *A Farewell to English*, The Gallery Press, Meath, 1978.
11. Brendan Kelly, *Hearing Voices: The History of Psychiatry in Ireland*, Dublin, Irish Academic, 2016, p. 139.
12. Ibid.
13. https://www.irishaid.ie/news-publications/tags/poverty/
14. Joe Lee, Professor for Irish Studies and Director of Glucksman House, at New York University. Interview with author, *Story of Ireland*, BBC 2, 2011.

Chapter 4: Her Wars
1. WS 688, Kate O'Callaghan, Dublin.
2. Patrick Pearse, *The Murder Machine*, Corpus of Electronic Texts, University College Cork, p. 6.
3. Lloyd-George speech at Carnarvon, 10 October 1920, *New York Times*.
4. Cited in J. W. Taylor, *Guilty but Insane. JC Bowen-Colthurst: Villain or Victim*. Cork, 2016.
5. Professor Mary McAuliffe, 'Cumann na mBan and the deaths at Gortaglanna, Knockanure, North Kerry, 12 May 1921', Dublin, May 2021, https://marymcauliffe.blog/2021/05/12/cumann-na-mban-and-the-deaths-at-gortaglanna-knockanure-north-kerry-may-12-1921-a-centenary-reflection/
6. WS 1013, Patrick McElligott.
7. Gobnait Ni Bhruadair, cited in Professor Mary McAuliffe, 'Cumann na mBan and the deaths at Gortaglanna, Knockanure, North Kerry, 12 May 1921', Dublin, May 2021.
8. Hannah Keane, Military Pensions Application File, MD 41314, BMH, Dublin.
9. Her employer, Edward J. Stack, reported NA: CO 762/100/15.
10. NA: CO 762/100/15.
11. Ibid.
12. WS 688, Kate O'Callaghan.
13. WS 544, Joseph O'Connor.

14. WS 444, Peter Kearney.
15. W. B. Yeats, *Nineteen Nineteen*, The Tower, 1928.
16. May Ahern, cited in Hannah Keane, Military Pensions Application File, MD41314, BMH, Dublin.
17. Ibid.
18. Fergal Keane, *Wounds*, William Collins, London, 2017, p. 290.
19. Wilfred Owen, 'Dulce et Decorum Est', *Poems*, Chatto and Windus, London, 1920.
20. May Ahern, cited in Hannah Keane, Military Pensions Application File, MD41314, BMH, Dublin.
21. W. U. Eckart (2017) 'The Soldier's Body in Gas Warfare: Trauma, Illness', *Rentennot*, 1915–1933, https://doi.org/10.1007/978-3-319-51664-6_12
22. Lt.-Col. Arthur A. Hanbury-Sparrow, *The land-locked lake: Impressions of active service in the European War*, London: Arthur Baker, 1932.
23. W. H. R. Rivers, 'On the Repression of War Experience', *Proceedings of the Royal Society of Medicine*, Vol. 11, Issue: Sect_Psych: 1–20, 1 April 1918.
24. O'Sullivan, Patricia, *St Finan's Hospital, Killarney: History of Mental Health in County Kerry*, www.stfinanshospital.com
25. Ibid.
26. Cited in David Cronin. 'Winston Churchill sent the Black and Tans to Palestine', *Irish Times*, 19 May 2017.
27. Cited in Hannah Keane, Military Pensions Application File, MD41314, BMH, Dublin.
28. Ibid.
29. Author interview.
30. Author interview.

Chapter 5: Hero Child

1. A. M. Leahy, *Heroic Romances of Ireland*, Vol. I, 1905, www.sacred-texts.com
2. Meg Jay, *Supernormal: Childhood Adversity and the Untold Story of Resilience*, Canongate, 2017, p. 106.
3. Freya McClements, 'Northern Ireland's Refugees Fifty Years On', *Irish Times*, 7 August 2021.
4. Pádraig Pearse, *Peace and The Gael*, 1915, Corpus of Electronic Texts, University College Cork, www.celt.ucc.ie
5. Cited in John Dorney, 'Events in Terenure in the Irish War of Independence and Civil War', *The Irish Story*, 9 September 2019.
6. See http://scoilbhride1917.ie/page/Stair-na-Scoile--Cead-Bliain-faoi-Bhlath/6838/Index.html

7. Patrick Pearse, *Óró, sé do bheatha bhaile*, 1914.

8. Geraldine Glover, 'The Hero Child in the Alcoholic Home', *The School Counsellor*, 41(3), 185–90. https://www.jstor.org/stable/23900659

Chapter 6: Reckonings

1. Alan Seeger, 'I Have a Rendezvous with Death', *A Treasury of War Poetry*, ed. George Herbert Clarke, 1917.

2. Kevin Carter, death note, cited in https://www.sahistory.org.za/dated-event/south-african-photojournalist-and-member-bang-bang-club-kevin-carter-commits-suicide

3. Desmond Tutu, foreword to *The Bang-Bang Club*, by Greg Marinovich, Joao Silva, Arrow Books, 2012, Kindle edn, p. 68.

4. Ibid.

Chapter 7: Believing

1. General Roméo Dallaire interviewed by Brian Bethune in *MacLean's* magazine, 21 October 2016: https://www.macleans.ca/culture/books/inside-romeo-dallaires-brutally-revealing-new-memoir/

2. Author interview.

3. *Judgement of the Trial Chamber in the case of ICTR v Nyiramasuhuko*, International Criminal Tribunal for Rwanda.

4. Author interview.

5. Summary of Judgement and Sentence. Prosecutor v. Nyiramasuhuko et al., Case No. ICTR-98-42-T, Judgement of the International Criminal Tribunal.

6. Ibid.

7. Cited by Thierry Cruvellier and Franck Petit, Diplomatique Judicaire Arusha, 10 November 2001.

8. Gilad Hirschberger, 'Collective Trauma and the Social Construction of Meaning', *Frontiers in Psychology*, 10 August 2018.

9. Author interview.

Chapter 8: Abandoned

1. Cheryl Ntakirutimana, 'Farewell', https://www.poetrysoup.com

2. Author interview.

3. Testimony of Sylvain Nsabimana, International Criminal Tribunal for Rwanda, 16 October 2006.

4. Author interview.

5. Author interview.

6. Author interview.

7. Author interview.

Chapter 9: Blackout Boy

1. Jon Loomis, 'Deer Hit', in *The Pleasure Principle*, Oberlin College Press, Field Poetry Series, Vol. 11, 2001.
2. Howard J. Edenberg, and Tatiana Foroud, Genetics and Alcoholism, *Nature Reviews. Gastroenterology & Hepatology*, Vol. 10,8 (2013): 487–94. doi:10.1038/nrgastro.2013.86
3. F. Scott Fitzgerald, *The Great Gatsby*, New York, Scribner's, 1925.
4. Stephen Spender, 'The War God' in 'Part Two: The Ironies of War', from *New Collected Poems*, Faber & Faber, 2004.

Chapter 10: The Fires Are Everywhere

1. Antoine de Saint-Exupéry, *The Little Prince*, p. 57, https://TheVirtualLibrary.org
2. Anton La Guardia, 'Airborne Adventurer Keeps Freetown Free', *Daily Telegraph*, 18 June 2000.
3. *The Law Reports of the Special Court for Sierra Leone, Vol. 3*, ed. Charles Chernor Jalloh, Simon M. Meisenberg, Brill Nijhof, Leiden – Boston, 2015.

Chapter 11: Terms of Surrender

1. Traditional ballad 'María Soliña', Ferreiro, C. E. and Paz Valverde E., *Vida e Morte*. Disques Alvarez, 1974.
2. Colm O Lochlainn, *Irish Street Ballads*, Constable & Co, Ltd., London, 1939.
3. Clare Campbell, *Out of It: How Cocaine Killed My Brother*, Hodder & Stoughton, London, 2007.

Chapter 12: Siege

1. Aeschylus, 'Agamemnon', *The Greek Plays*, eds Mary Lefkowitz and James Romm, Ballantine Books (reprint edition 2015), New York, p. 10.
2. Raymond Whitaker, 'Robert Fisk Beaten By Mob', *Independent*, 9 December 2001.
3. Fergal Keane, *All of These People*, HarperCollins, London, 2005, p. 379.
4. Fergal Keane, in *Love Poet, Carpenter*, Enitharmon Press, London, 2009, p. 75.
5. Michael Longley, 'All of These People', *Collected Poems*, 2007.
6. Human Rights Watch, 'Repression of the Popular Protests in Burma', 2007.

Chapter 13: Old Ground

1. David Orr, Letter to Raymond Mbaraga, genocide survivor, 16 February 2021: https://www.newtimes.co.rw/news/genocide-letter-man-who-dared-tell-truth
2. Susan Sontag, *Regarding the Pain of Others*, Penguin, 2003, pp. 28, 62.
3. Beata Umubyeyi Mairesse, *All Your Children, Scattered*, Europa Editions, 2022.
4. Linda Melvern, 'History? This Film is Fiction', *Guardian*, 18 March 2006.
5. Radio des Mille Collines broadcast, 24 April 1994.
6. Daphna Canetti, Eran Halperin, Agneta Fischer, Alba Jasini, 'Why We Hate', *Emotion Review*, October 2014.
7. Author interview.
8. Author interview.
9. Author interview.
10. Author interview.
11. Author interview.

Chapter 14: Trials

1. John Milton, *Paradise Lost*, ed. Robert Vaughan, Cassell and Co., London, 1894 (Digital edition 2006), Book 1, p. 3.
2. Roméo Dallaire, *Shake Hands with the Devil*, Random House, 2003, p. 289.
3. Bessel van der Kolk, *The Body Keeps the Score*, Penguin Books, 2014, p. 253.
4. https://womenstherapyinstitute.com/guilt-is-grandiose
5. Michael Ignatieff, from foreword to Simon Norfolk, *For Most of It I Have No Words*, Dewi Lewis Books, 1998.
6. See https://www.ptsd.va.gov/understand/what/avoidance.asp

Chapter 15: East

1. Author interview.
2. 'Report of the Joint Investigation Team into the shooting down of Malaysian Airlines Flight MH17', August 2015.
3. Ibid.
4. Anton Chekhov, from *The Steppe and Other Stories, 1887–91*, Penguin Books, 2001, p. 7.
5. Susan Sontag, *Regarding the Pain of Others*, Penguin Books, 2004, p. 100.

Chapter 16: Trip Wires
1. Serhiy Zhadan, 'So I'll Talk About It', translated by John Hennessy and Ostap Kin, https://www.asymptotejournal.com/poetry/serhiy-zhadan-four-poems/
2. Interviews with author.
3. Anna Akhmatova, 'White Flock', 1917, translated by Andrey Kneller.

Chapter 17: Breakdown
1. Khalil Gibran, 'Fear', 1923.
2. Author interview.
3. Alexander Dumas, *The Count of Monte Cristo*, p. 1067, electronic edition, http://www.literaturepage.com
4. Edward Thomas quoted in Helen Thomas to Robert Frost, March 1917, Dartmouth College Library Bulletin, 1990.
5. Edward Thomas, 'The Owl', 1915, *Selected Poems*, ed. Matthew Hollis, London, 2011.

Chapter 18: For Fear of a Dream
1. Michael Flack, 'Terezín', 1944, United States Holocaust Memorial Museum Collection, gift of Anna Hanusová-Flachová.
2. 'Huon of Bordeaux', trans. John Bourchier Berners, retold by Robert Steele, George Allen, 1895.
3. Interview with author.
4. Ibid.
5. Ibid.
6. Charlotte Delbo, 'Prayer to the Living to Forgive Them for Being Alive', in *Auschwitz and After*, trans. Rosette C. Lamont, Yale University Press, 2014, p. 230.

Chapter 19: Gathering In
1. Hart Crane, 'The Broken Tower'. *The Complete Poems of Hart Crane: The Centennial Edition*, Liveright Publishing, 1932, pp. 160–1.
2. Interview with author.
3. Interview with author.
4. Ibid.
5. Ibid.
6. Ibid.
7. Ibid.
8. Raymond Carver, 'Where Water Comes Together With Other Water', in *All of Us: The Collected Poems*, Vintage, 2000.